Shaping
History
Through
PRAYER
and **FASTING**

Shaping History Through PRAYER and FASTING

Derek Prince

Whitaker House

Unless otherwise indicated, all Scripture quotations are taken from the *King James Version* (KJV) of the Bible.

Scripture quotations identified (RSV) are from the *Revised Standard Version* of the Bible, © 1946 and 1952.

Scripture quotations identified (NEB) are from *The New English Bible, New Testament, Second Edition,* © 1961, 1970 by The Delegates of the Oxford University Press and the Syndics of the Cambridge University Press. Used by permission.

Scripture quotations identified (PHILLIPS) are from *The New Testament in Modern English,* translated by J. B. Phillips, © 1958, 1959, 1960, 1972 by J. B. Phillips, and © 1947, 1952, 1955, 1957 by The MacMillan Company. Used by permission.

Excerpts from *Of Plymouth Plantation* by William Bradford, edited by Samuel Eliot Morison, © 1952 by Random House, Inc. Used by permission.

Excerpts from *A Christian History of the Constitution* by Verna M. Hall, © 1960 by The American Constitution Press, San Francisco, California.

SHAPING HISTORY THROUGH PRAYER AND FASTING

Derek Prince Ministries - International
1800 East Associates Lane
Charlotte, NC 28217

ISBN: 0-88368-339-3
Printed in the United States of America
Copyright © 1973 by Derek Prince

Whitaker House
580 Pittsburgh Street
Springdale, PA 15144

Contents

By The President of
The United States of America:

A Proclamation

For a Day of National Humiliation Fasting and Prayer

Whereas, the Senate of the United States, devoutly recognizing the Supreme Authority and Just Government of Almighty God, in all the affairs of men and of nations, has, by a resolution, requested the President to designate and set apart a day for National prayer and humiliation:

And whereas, it is the duty of nations, as well as of men, to own their dependence upon the overruling power of God, to confess their sins and transgressions, in humble sorrow, yet with assured hope that genuine repentance will lead to mercy and pardon; and to recognize the sublime truth, announced in the Holy Scriptures and proven by all history, that those nations only are blessed whose God is the Lord:

And, insomuch as we know that, by His divine law, nations, like individuals, are subjected to punishments and chastisements in this world, may we not justly fear that the awful calamity of civil war, which now desolates the land, may be but a punishment inflicted upon us for our presumptuous sins, to the needful end of our national reformation as a whole People? We have been the recipients of the choicest bounties of Heaven. We have been preserved, these many years, in peace and prosperity. We have grown in numbers, wealth, and power as no other nation has ever grown. But we have forgotten God. We have forgotten the gracious hand which preserved us in peace, and multiplied and enriched and strengthened us; and we have vainly imagined, in the deceitfulness of our hearts, that all these blessings were produced by some superior wisdom and virtue of our own. Intoxicated with unbroken success, we have become too self-sufficient to feel the necessity of redeeming and preserving grace, too proud to pray to the God that made us! It behooves us, then, to humble ourselves before the offended Power, to confess our national sins, and to pray for clemency and forgiveness.

Now, therefore, in compliance with the request, and fully concurring in the views of the Senate, I do, by this my proclamation, designate and set apart Thursday, the 30th day of April, 1863, as a day of national humiliation, fasting, and prayer. And I do hereby request all the People to abstain on that day from their ordinary secular pursuits, and to unite, at their several places of public worship and their respective homes, in keeping the day holy to the Lord, and devoted to the humble discharge of the religious duties proper to that solemn occasion.

All this being done, in sincerity and truth, let us then rest humbly in the hope authorized by the Divine teachings, that the united cry of the Nation will be heard on high, and answered with blessings, no less than the pardon of our national sins, and restoration of our now divided and suffering *country, to its former happy condition of unity and peace.*

In witness whereof, I have hereunto set my hand, and caused the seal of the United States to be affixed.

Done at the city of Washington this thirtieth day of March, in the year of our Lord one thousand eight hundred and sixty-three, and of the Independence of the United States the eighty-seventh.

Abraham Lincoln

By the President:
WILLIAM H. SEWARD, *Secretary of State*

The above proclamation is preserved in the Library of Congress as Appendix no. 19 in volume 12 of the United States At Large. It was initiated by a resolution of the United States Senate, and was officially declared by President Lincoln on March 30, 1863.

Its message contains two related themes which challenge our careful consideration.

First, the proclamation acknowledges the unique blessings enjoyed by the United States, but suggests that these blessings have brought about an attitude of pride and self-sufficiency which are the root causes of a grave national crisis. Some of the phrases could apply with equal force to the condition of the nation today: "We have grown in numbers, wealth, and power as no other nation has ever grown....We have vainly imagined, in the deceitfulness of our hearts, that all these blessings were produced by some superior wisdom and virtue of our own....We have become too self-sufficient...too proud to pray to the God that made us!"

Second, the proclamation unequivocally acknowledges "the overruling power of God" in the affairs of men and nations. It indicates that behind the political, economic, and military forces of history, there are divine spiritual laws at work; and that by acknowledging and submitting to these laws a nation may change its destiny, averting threatened disaster and regaining true peace and prosperity. In particular, the proclamation sets forth one specific, practical way in which a nation may invoke on its own behalf "the overruling power of God"—that is, by united prayer and fasting.

The author of this proclamation, Abraham Lincoln, is generally regarded, both by Americans and by the world at large, as one of the shrewdest and most enlightened of American presidents. He was a man of sincere faith and deep convictions, but he never sought membership in any of the Christian denominations of his day. In no sense could he be considered as unbalanced or extreme in his religious views. Further, this proclamation was not merely the product of Lincoln's private convictions. It was requested by a resolution of the entire United States Senate.

How shall we assess the deep and unanimous convictions of men of this caliber? Shall we dismiss them as irrelevant or out-of-date? To do this would be merely the mark of unreasoning prejudice.

Rather, we owe it to ourselves to give honest and careful consideration to this proclamation and the issues which it raises. Is there a divine Power that overrules the destinies of nations? Can this power effectively be invoked by prayer and fasting?

It is to the examination of these questions that this book is devoted. An answer will be offered from four main sources: first, the teaching of Scripture; second, events of world history during or after World War II; third, the annals of American history; fourth, records of personal experience in the realm of prayer and fasting.

Derek Prince

1

The Salt of the Earth

"Ye are the salt of the earth."
—Matthew 5:13

Jesus is speaking to His disciples—to all of us, that is, who acknowledge the authority of His teaching. He compares our function on the earth to that of salt. His meaning becomes clear when we consider two familiar uses of salt in relation to food.

Salt Gives Flavor

First of all, salt gives flavor. Food which in itself is unappetizing becomes tasty and acceptable when seasoned with salt. In Job 6:6 this is put in the form of a rhetorical question: *"Can that which is unsavory be eaten without salt?*" It is the presence of salt that makes the difference, causing us to enjoy food which we would otherwise have refused to eat. As Christians, our function is to give flavor to the earth. The one who enjoys this flavor is God. Our presence makes the earth acceptable to God. Our presence commends the earth to God's mercy. Without us, there would be nothing to make the earth acceptable to God. But because we are here, God continues to deal with the earth in grace and mercy rather than in wrath and judgment. It is our presence that makes the difference.

This principle is vividly illustrated in the account of Abraham's intercession on behalf of Sodom, as recorded in Genesis 18:16-33. The Lord has told Abraham that He is on His way to Sodom to see if that city's wickedness has come to the point where judgment can no longer be withheld. Abraham then walks with the Lord on the way toward Sodom and reasons with Him about the principles of His judgment.

First, Abraham establishes one principle that is the basis for all that follows: **It is never the will of God that the judgment due to the wicked should come upon the righteous**. *"Wilt thou also destroy the righteous with the wicked?"* (v. 23) Abraham asks. *"That be far from thee to do after this*

*manner, to slay the righteous with the wicked:
and that the righteous should be as the wicked,
that be far from thee: Shall not the Judge of all
the earth do right?"* (v. 25).

The Lord makes clear in the ensuing conversation that He accepts the principle stated
by Abraham. How important it is that all believers understand this! If we have been made
righteous by faith in Christ, and if we are leading lives that truly express our faith, then it is
never God's will that we be included in the
judgments which He brings upon the wicked.

Unfortunately, Christians often do not
understand this because they fail to distinguish between two situations which outwardly
may appear similar, but which in reality are
completely different in nature and cause. On
the one hand, there is persecution for the sake
of righteousness. On the other hand, there is
God's judgment upon the wicked. The difference between these two situations is brought
out by the following contrasted statements:
Persecution comes from the wicked upon the
righteous; but judgment comes from God, who
is righteous, upon the wicked. Thus, persecution for righteousness and judgment for wickedness are opposite to each other in their
origins, their purposes and their results.

The Bible plainly warns that Christians
must expect to suffer persecution. In the

Sermon on the Mount, Jesus says to His disciples: *"Blessed are they which are persecuted for righteousness' sake: for theirs is the kingdom of heaven. Blessed are ye when men shall revile you, and persecute you, and shall say all manner of evil against you falsely, for my sake"* (Matthew 5:10-11). Paul writes likewise to Timothy: *"Yea, and all that will live godly in Christ Jesus shall suffer persecution"* (2 Timothy 3:12). Christians must therefore be prepared to endure persecution for their faith and their way of life, and even to count this as a privilege.

But by the same token Christians should never be included in God's judgments upon the wicked. This principle is stated many times in Scripture. In 1 Corinthians 11:32, Paul writes to his fellow believers, and he says, *"But when we* [Christians] *are judged, we are chastened of the Lord that we should not be condemned with the world."* This demonstrates that there is a difference between God's dealings with believers and His dealings with the world. As believers, we may expect to experience God's chastening. If we submit to the chastening and set our lives in order, then we are not subject to the judgments that come upon unbelievers, or the world in general. The very purpose of God's chastening us as believers is to preserve us from undergoing His judgments upon unbelievers.

In Psalm 91:7-8, the psalmist gives this promise to the believer: *"A thousand shall fall at thy side, and ten thousand at thy right hand; but it shall not come nigh thee. Only with thine eyes shalt thou behold and see the reward of the wicked."* Here again the principle is seen. Whatever judgment comes as *"the reward of the wicked"* (that which the wicked justly deserve) should never fall upon the righteous. No matter if God strikes the wicked on every side, the righteous in the midst of it all will not be harmed.

In Exodus chapters 7 through 12, it is recorded that God brought ten judgments of ever-increasing severity upon the Egyptians because they refused to listen to His prophets Moses and Aaron. Throughout all this, God's people Israel dwelt in the midst of Egypt, but not one of the ten judgments touched them. In Exodus 11:7, the reason is graphically stated: *"But against any of the children of Israel shall not a dog move his tongue, against man or beast: that ye may know that the Lord doth put a difference between the Egyptians and Israel."* Judgment did not come upon Israel because the Lord *"put a difference"* between His own people and the people of Egypt. Even the dogs of Egypt had to acknowledge this difference! And the difference is valid to this day.

Continuing his conversation with the Lord concerning Sodom, Abraham attempts to ascertain the least number of righteous persons needed to preserve the whole city from judgment. He begins with fifty. Then with a remarkable combination of reverence and perseverance, he works his way down to ten. The Lord finally assures Abraham that if He finds only ten righteous persons in Sodom, He will spare the whole city for the sake of those ten.

What was the population of Sodom? It would be difficult to arrive at an exact estimate. However, there are figures available for certain other cities of ancient Palestine that provide a standard of comparison. In Abraham's day the walls of Jericho enclosed an area of about seven or eight acres. This would provide dwelling space for a minimum of five thousand persons or a maximum of ten thousand. But Jericho was not a large city by the standards of its day. The largest city of that period was Hazor, which covered about 175 acres and had a population estimated at between forty and fifty thousand. Later, in the period of Joshua, we are told that the total population of Ai was twelve thousand persons (Joshua 8:25). The Bible record seems to indicate that Sodom was a more important city in its day than Ai.

Taking these other cities into account, we could say that the population of Sodom in Abraham's day was probably not less than ten thousand. God assured Abraham that ten righteous persons could by their very presence preserve a city of at least ten thousand. This gives a ratio of one to a thousand. The same ratio of *"one among a thousand"* is given in Job 33:23 and in Ecclesiastes 7:28, and both these passages suggest that the *"one"* is a person of outstanding righteousness, while all the remainder fall below God's standards.

It is easy to extend this ratio indefinitely. The presence of ten righteous persons can preserve a community of ten thousand. The presence of a hundred righteous persons can preserve a community of one hundred thousand. The presence of one thousand righteous persons can preserve a community of one million. How many righteous persons are needed to preserve a nation as large as the United States, with an estimated population of nearly 250,000,000? About 250,000 persons.

These figures are evocative. Does Scripture give us grounds to believe that, for example, a quarter of a million truly righteous persons, scattered as grains of salt across the United States, would suffice to preserve the entire nation from God's judgment and to ensure the continuance of His grace and mercy? It would be foolish to claim that such estimates are exact. Nevertheless, the Bible definitely establishes the general principle that the presence of righteous believers is the decisive factor in God's dealings with a community.

To illustrate this principle, Jesus uses the metaphor of *"salt."* In 2 Corinthians 5:20, Paul uses a different metaphor to convey the same truth: *"We are ambassadors for Christ."* What are ambassadors? They are persons sent forth in an official capacity by a nation's government to represent that government in the territory of another nation. Their authority is not measured by their own personal abilities, but is in direct proportion to the authority of the government which they represent.

In Philippians 3:20, Paul specifies the government which, as Christians, we represent. He says, *"Our conversation* [literally, our citizenship] *is in heaven."* Two translations render this, *"We are citizens of heaven"* (PHILLIPS and NEB). Thus our position on earth is that of ambassadors representing heaven's government. We have no authority to act on our own, but as long as we carefully obey the directions of our government, the entire might and authority of heaven are behind every word that we speak and every move that we make.

Before one government declares war on another, its usual action of final warning is to withdraw its ambassadors. While we are left on earth as heaven's ambassadors, our presence guarantees a continuance of God's forbearance and mercy toward the earth. But when heaven's ambassadors are finally withdrawn, there will then be nothing left to hold back the full outpouring of divine wrath and judgment upon the earth.

This leads us to a second effect of the presence of Christians as *"the salt of the earth."*

Salt Restrains Corruption

A second function of salt in relation to food is to restrain the process of corruption. In the days before artificial refrigeration, sailors who took meat on long voyages used salt as a preservative. The process of corruption was already at work before the meat was salted. Salting did not abolish the corruption, but it held it in check for the duration of the voyage, so that the sailors could continue to eat the meat long after it would otherwise have become inedible.

Our presence on the earth as Christ's disciples operates like the salt in the meat. The process of sin's corruption is already at work.

This is manifested in every area of human activity—moral, religious, social, political. We cannot abolish the corruption which is already there, but we can hold it in check long enough for God's purposes of grace and mercy to be fully worked out. Then, when our influence is no longer felt, corruption will come to its climax, and the result will be total degradation.

This illustration from the power of salt to restrain corruption explains Paul's teaching in 2 Thessalonians 2:3-12. Paul warns that human wickedness will come to its climax in the person of a world ruler supernaturally empowered and directed by Satan himself. Paul calls this ruler *"the man of sin"* (more literally, *"the man of lawlessness"*), and *"the son of perdition"* (v. 3). In 1 John 2:18, he is called *"antichrist."* In Revelation 13:4, he is called *"the beast."* This ruler will actually claim to be God and will demand universal worship.

Emergence of this satanic ruler is inevitable. Paul says with certainty, *"Then shall that Wicked* [lawless one] *be revealed"* (2 Thessalonians 2:8). Paul also declares in the same verse that the true Christ Himself will be the one to administer final judgment upon this false Christ: *"whom the Lord shall consume with the spirit* [breath] *of his mouth, and shall destroy with the brightness of his coming."*

Unfortunately some preachers have used this teaching about antichrist to instill into Christians an attitude of passivity and fatalism. "Antichrist is coming," they have said, "Things are getting worse and worse. There is nothing we can do about it." As a result, Christians have all too often sat back with folded hands, in pious dismay, and watched the ravages of Satan proceed unchecked all around them.

This attitude of passivity and fatalism is as tragic as it is unscriptural. It is true that antichrist must eventually emerge. But it is far from true that there is nothing to be done about him in the meanwhile. To this present moment there is a force at work in the world that challenges, resists and restrains the spirit of antichrist. The work of this force is described by Paul in 2 Thessalonians 2:6-7. Freely rendered in modern English, these verses might read as follows: *"And now you know what holds him in check until he is revealed in his time. For the secret power of lawlessness is already at work: only he who now holds him in check will continue to do so until he is withdrawn or taken out of the midst"* (author's paraphrase).

This restraining power, which at present holds back the full and final emergence of antichrist, is the personal presence of the Holy

Spirit within the church. This becomes clear as we follow the unfolding revelation of Scripture concerning the Person and the work of the Holy Spirit. At the very beginning of the Bible, in Genesis 1:2, we are told, *"the Spirit of God moved upon the face of the waters."* From then on throughout the Old Testament, we find frequent references to the activity of the Holy Spirit in the earth. However, at the close of His earthly ministry, Jesus promised His disciples that the Holy Spirit would shortly come to them in a new way, different from anything that had ever taken place on earth up to that time.

In John 14:16-17 Jesus gives this promise: *"And I will pray the Father, and he shall give you another Comforter, that he may abide with you for ever; Even the Spirit of truth* [a title of the Holy Spirit]*...for he dwelleth with you, and shall be in you."* We may paraphrase this promise of Jesus as follows: "I have been with you in personal presence three-and-a-half years, and I am now about to leave you. After I have gone, another Person will come to take my place. This Person is the Holy Spirit. When He comes, He will remain with you for ever."

In John 16:6-7, Jesus repeats His promise: *"But because I have said these things unto you, sorrow hath filled your heart. Nevertheless I tell you the truth; it is expedient for you that I go away: for if I go not away, the Comforter will not come unto you; but if I depart, I will send him unto you."* The picture is clear. There is to be an exchange of Persons. Jesus will depart, but in His place another Person will come. This other Person is the Comforter, the Holy Spirit.

In John 16:12-13, Jesus returns to this theme for the third time: *"I have yet many things to say unto you, but ye cannot bear them now. Howbeit when he, the Spirit of truth, is come, he will guide you into all truth."* In the original Greek text, the pronoun *"he"* is in the masculine gender, but the noun *"Spirit"* is neuter. This grammatical conflict of genders brings out the dual nature of the Holy Spirit—both personal and impersonal. This agrees with the language used by Paul in 2 Thessalonians chapter 2 concerning the power which holds back the emergence of antichrist. In verse 6 Paul says, *"What is restraining him"* (RSV), and in verse 7 he says, *"He who now restrains him"* (RSV). This similarity of expression confirms the identification of this restraining power with the Holy Spirit.

The exchange of persons promised by Jesus was effected in two stages: first, the ascension of Jesus into heaven; then, ten days later, the descent of the Holy Spirit on the day of Pentecost. At this point in history the Holy

Spirit descended as a Person from heaven and took up His residence on earth. He is now the personal Representative of the Godhead resident on earth. His actual dwelling place is the body of true believers, called collectively *"the church."* To this body of believers Paul says in 1 Corinthians 3:16: *"Know ye not that ye are the temple of God, and that the Spirit of God dwelleth in you?"*

The great ministry of the Holy Spirit within the church is to prepare a completed body for Christ. After completion, this body will in turn be presented to Christ as a bride is presented to a bridegroom. As soon as this ministry of the Holy Spirit within the church is finished, He will again be withdrawn from the earth, taking with Him the completed body of Christ. Thus we may fill out Paul's statement in 2 Thessalonians 2:7 as follows: *"He* [the Holy Spirit] *who now holds him* [the antichrist] *in check will continue to do so until he be withdrawn."*

The opposition between the Holy Spirit and the spirit of antichrist is described also in 1 John 4:3-4: *"And every spirit that confesseth not that Jesus Christ is come in the flesh is not of God: and this is that spirit of antichrist, whereof ye have heard that it should come, and even now already is it in the world. Ye are of God, little children, and have overcome them:*

because greater is he that is in you, that he that is in the world."

In the world is the spirit of antichrist, working toward the emergence of antichrist himself. In the disciples of Christ is the Holy Spirit, holding back the emergence of antichrist. Therefore the disciples who are indwelled by the Holy Spirit act as a barrier, holding back the climax of lawlessness and the final emergence of antichrist. Only when the Holy Spirit, together with the completed body of Christ's disciples, is withdrawn from the earth, will the forces of lawlessness be able to proceed without restraint to the culmination of their purposes in antichrist. Meanwhile, it is both the privilege and the responsibility of Christ's disciples, by the power of the Holy Spirit, to *"overcome"* the forces of antichrist and to hold them in check.

The Consequences of Failure

As the salt of earth, then, we who are Christ's disciples have two primary responsibilities. First, by our presence we commend the earth to God's continuing grace and mercy. Second, by the power of the Holy Spirit within us, we hold in check the forces of corruption and lawlessness until God's appointed time.

In fulfilling these responsibilities, the church stands as the barrier to the accomplishment of Satan's supreme ambition, which is to gain dominion over the whole earth. This explains why Paul says in 2 Thessalonians 2:3 that there must be *"a falling away first, before the man of sin* [antichrist] *can be revealed."* The world translated *"falling away"* is literally *apostasy*—that is, a departure from the faith. So long as the church stands firm and uncompromising in its faith, it has the power to hold back the final manifestation of antichrist. Satan himself fully understands this, and therefore his primary objective is to undermine the faith and righteousness of the church. Once he achieves this, the barrier to his purposes is removed, and the way is open for him to gain both spiritual and political control over the whole earth.

Suppose that Satan succeeds, because we, as Christians, fail to fulfill our responsibilities. What then? Jesus Himself gives us the answer. We become *"salt that has lost its savor."* He warns us of the fate that awaits such savorless salt: *"It is thenceforth good for nothing, but to be cast out, and to be trodden under foot of men"* (Matthew 5:13).

"Good for nothing!" That is severe condemnation indeed. What follows? We are *"cast out,"* or rejected by God. Then we are *"trodden*

under foot of men." Men become the instruments of God's judgment upon a saltless, apostate church. If we in the church fail to hold back the forces of wickedness, our judgment is to be handed over to those very forces.

The alternatives that confront us are clearly presented by Paul in Romans 12:21: *"Be not overcome with evil, but overcome evil with good."* There are only two choices: either to overcome, or to be overcome. There is no middle way, no third course open to us. We may use the good that God has put at our disposal to overcome the evil that confronts us. But if we fail to do this, then that very evil will in turn overcome us.

This message applies with special urgency to those of us who live in lands where we still enjoy liberty to proclaim and to practice our Christian faith. In many lands today Christians have lost this liberty. At the same time multiplying millions in those lands have been systematically indoctrinated to hate and to despise Christianity and all that it stands for. To people thus indoctrinated there could be no greater satisfaction than to trample under their feet those Christians who are not already under their yoke.

If we heed the warning of Jesus, and fulfill our functions as salt in the earth, we have the power to prevent this. But if we default from our responsibilities and suffer the judgment that follows, the bitterest reflection of all will be this: **It need never have happened!**

2

A Kingdom of Priests

God has vested in us—His believing people on earth—authority by which we may determine the destinies of nations and governments. He expects us to use our authority both for His glory and for our own good. If we fail to do so, we are answerable for the consequences. Such is the message of Scripture, unfolded both by precept and by pattern. It is confirmed by the personal experience of many believers and is written across the pages of the history of whole nations. In later chapters we will examine specific instances of this, taken from the events of recent world history and also from the annals of American history. But first, in this chapter, we will study the scriptural basis of this authority.

God's Words in Man's Mouth

An outstanding example is provided by the career of the prophet Jeremiah. In the opening ten verses of the first chapter of Jeremiah, God declares that He has set Jeremiah apart *"as a prophet unto the nations"* (1:5). Jeremiah in response protests his inability to fulfill this role, saying, *"I cannot speak: for I am* [only a youth]." However, God reaffirms His call in stronger terms and concludes by saying, *"See, I have this day set thee over the nations and over the kingdoms, to root out, and to pull down, and to destroy, and to throw down, to build, and to plant"* (v. 10).

What an exalted position for a young man, to be *"set over the nations and over the kingdoms."* This is authority on a higher plane than the normal forces that shape secular politics. To judge by outward appearances, the subsequent career of Jeremiah gave little indication of such authority. On the contrary, his message was almost universally rejected, and he himself was continually subjected to indignity and persecution. For several months he languished in prison, and at various times he was at the point of death, either by execution or by starvation.

Yet the course of history has vindicated the authority of Jeremiah and his message. His prophetic messages unfolded the destinies of Israel and of nearly all the surrounding nations in the Middle East, as well as those of nations in other areas of the earth. Twenty-five hundred years have passed. In the light of history it is now possible to make an objective evaluation. Throughout all the intervening centuries the destiny of every one of those nations has followed precisely the course foretold by Jeremiah. The more closely we compare their subsequent histories with the prophecies of Jeremiah, the more exactly do we find them to correspond. Thus Jeremiah was in very fact *"set over those nations and over those kingdoms,"* and by the prophecies that he uttered he became the actual arbiter of their destinies.

What was the basis of such tremendous authority? The answer is found in Jeremiah 1:9: *"And the Lord said unto me, Behold, I have put my words in thy mouth."* The authority lay in God's words, imparted to Jeremiah. Because the words that Jeremiah uttered were not his own, but those that God gave him, they were just as effective in Jeremiah's mouth as they would have been in the mouth of God Himself. In all earth's affairs the last word is with God. At times, however, God causes this word to be spoken through the lips of a human believer. Such a word may be spoken publicly in prophecy, or in the authoritative exposition of Scripture. More often, perhaps, it is spoken within a prayer closet, in petition or in intercession.

It is important to observe that Jeremiah stood in a twofold relationship to the secular government of his day. On the natural plane, as a citizen of Judah, he was in subjection to the government of his nation, represented by the king and the princes. In no sense did he preach or practice political subversion or anarchy. Nor did he ever seek to evade or to resist decrees made by the government concerning him, even though these were at times arbitrary and unjust. Yet on the spiritual plane to which God elevated him through his prophetic ministry, Jeremiah exercised authority over the very rulers to whom he was in subjection on the natural plane.

Sharing the Throne with Christ

Jeremiah's career illustrates a principle which is more fully unfolded in the New Testament: **Every Christian has dual citizenship.** By natural birth he is a citizen of an earthly nation, and he is subject to all the ordinances and requirements of his nation's lawful government. But by spiritual rebirth, through faith in Christ, he is also a citizen of God's heavenly kingdom. This is the basis of

Paul's statement, already referred to in our previous chapter: *"We...are citizens of heaven"* (Philippians 3:20 NEB).

As a citizen of heaven, the Christian is subject to the laws of the heavenly kingdom, but he is also entitled to share in its authority. This is the kingdom of which David speaks in Psalm 103:19: *"The Lord hath prepared his throne in the heavens; and his kingdom ruleth over all."* God's kingdom is supreme over all other kingdoms and over all other forces at work on earth. It is God's purpose to share the authority of His kingdom with His believing people. In Luke 12:32, Jesus assures His disciples, *"Fear not, little flock; for it is your Father's good pleasure to give you the kingdom."* The comfort of this assurance does not depend upon the strength or numbers of the flock, for it is a *"little flock,"* a company of *"sheep in the midst of wolves"* (Matthew 10:16). The certainty that the kingdom belongs to us is founded on the good pleasure of the Father, *"the purpose of him who worketh all things after the counsel of his own will"* (Ephesians 1:11).

As Christians, our position in God's kingdom is determined by our relationship to Christ. Paul explains this in Ephesians 2:4-6, which is rendered in the New English Bible: *"But God, rich in mercy, for the great love he bore us, brought us to life with Christ even when we were dead in our sins; it is by his grace you are saved. And in union with Christ Jesus he raised us up and enthroned us with him in the heavenly realms."*

God's grace identifies us with Christ in three successive phases. First, we are *"brought to life,"* or *"made alive."* We share Christ's life. Second, we are *"raised up,"* as Christ was raised up, from the tomb. We share Christ's resurrection. Third, we are *"enthroned"* in the heavenly kingdom. We share Christ's kingly authority on the throne. None of this is in the future. It is all stated in the past tense, as a fact already accomplished. Each of these three phases is made possible, not by our own efforts or merits, but solely by accepting in faith our union with Christ.

In Ephesians 1:20-21, Paul describes the position of supreme authority to which Christ has been exalted by the Father: *"when he raised him from the dead, when he enthroned him at his right hand in the heavenly realms, far above all government and authority, all power and dominion, and any title or sovereignty that can be named"* (NEB). Christ's authority at God's right hand does not necessarily set aside all other forms of authority or government, but it takes preeminence over them. The same truth is expressed by the title twice given to Christ in the Book of Revelation: *"King of kings and Lord of lords"* (Revelation 17:14; 19:16). Christ is the supreme Ruler over all rulers and Governor over all governments. This is the position on the throne which He shares with His believing people.

How shall we comprehend the magnitude of what is thus made available to us? The answer is given in Paul's prayer in the preceding verses of Ephesians chapter 1:

> *That the God of our Lord Jesus Christ, the Father of glory, may give you a spirit of wisdom and revelation in the knowledge of him, having the eyes of your heart enlightened, that you may know...what is the immeasurable greatness of his power in us who believe, according to the working of his great might which he accomplished in Christ when he raised him from the dead and made him sit at his right hand in the heavenly places.* (Ephesians 1:17-20 RSV)

This revelation cannot come by natural reasoning or by sense knowledge. It comes only by the Holy Spirit. He is the one who *"enlightens the eyes of our heart"* and shows us two interwoven truths: first, that Christ's authority is now supreme over the universe; second, that the same power that raised Christ to that position of authority now works also *"in us who believe."*

In 1 Corinthians chapter 2, Paul further explains these truths which are revealed to Christians only by the Holy Spirit. He says, *"But we impart a secret and hidden wisdom of God, which God decreed before the ages for our glorification. None of the rulers of this age understood this; for if they had, they would not have crucified the Lord of glory"* (vv. 7-8 RSV). This *"secret and hidden wisdom"* reveals Christ as *"Lord of glory."* It is *"for our glorification,"* for it shows us that in our union with Him we share His glory.

Paul continues, *"But, as it is written, 'What no eye has seen, nor ear heard, nor the heart of man conceived, what God has prepared for those who love him' God has revealed to us through the Spirit"* (vv. 9-10 RSV). Paul again emphasizes that knowledge of this kind is not imparted through the senses, nor is it forthcoming out of the inner resources of man's reason or imagination, except as these are illuminated by the Holy Spirit.

In verse 12, Paul sums this up: *"Now we have received, not the spirit of the world, but the spirit which is of God; that we might know the things that are freely given to us of God."* One of the things thus given to us is our position in Christ at God's right hand. Paul here contrasts two sources of knowledge. *"The spirit of the world"* shows us the things of this world. Through this we understand our earthly citizenship, with all its rights and responsibilities. But *"the Spirit which is of God"* reveals to us the kingdom of Christ and our place in it. Through this we understand our rights and responsibilities as citizens of heaven.

If, at times, our position with Christ on the throne seems remote or unreal, the reason is simple: We have not received the revelation which the Holy Spirit, through the Scriptures, makes available to us. Without this revelation we can neither understand nor enjoy the benefits of our heavenly citizenship. Instead of reigning as kings, we find ourselves still toiling as slaves.

From Slaves to Kings

From the beginning it was God's purpose to share with man His dominion over the earth. In Genesis 1:26, the initial purpose of man's creation is stated: *"And God said, Let us make man in our image after our likeness: and let them* [the human race] *have dominion... over all the earth."* Because of disobedience, Adam and his descendants forfeited their position of dominion. Instead of reigning in obedience as kings, they were subjugated as slaves to sin and to Satan.

However, the dominion that was lost to the whole race through Adam is restored to the believer in Christ. *"For if by one man's offense* [that is, the offense of Adam] *death reigned by one; much more they which receive abundance of grace and of the gift of righteousness shall reign in life by one, Jesus Christ"* (Romans 5:17). The consequences of Adam's disobedience and of Christ's obedience are both already manifested in this present life. Death reigns now over unbelievers. Likewise believers reign now in life by Christ. Through our union with Christ we have already been raised up to share the throne with Him, and we are reigning there with Him now.

God's purpose in man's redemption reflects His original purpose in man's creation. God's redeeming grace lifts man from his position of slavery and restores him to his position of dominion. In the Old Testament, this is demonstrated in the deliverance of Israel from the slavery of Egypt. In Exodus 19:6, God declares to Israel the purpose for which He has redeemed them: *"And ye shall be unto me a kingdom of priests, and a holy nation."* *"A kingdom of priests"* speaks of dominion restored—kingship in place of slavery. God offered Israel a double privilege: to minister as priests and to reign as kings. As we shall see in later chapters of this book, some of the great saints of Israel, such as Daniel, entered into this high calling. For the most part, however, the nation failed to accept God's gracious promises.

In the New Testament, to those redeemed by faith in Christ, God renews the calling that He originally gave to Israel. In 1 Peter 2:5, Christians are called *"an holy priesthood."* As priests of the New Testament, their ministry is *"to offer up spiritual sacrifices, acceptable to God by Jesus Christ."* The *"spiritual sacrifices"* offered up by Christians are the various forms of prayer—particularly worship and intercession. Then, in 1 Peter 2:9, Christians are further called *"a royal* [or kingly] *priesthood."* The phrase *"a royal priesthood"* exactly corresponds *to "a kingdom of priests"* in Exodus 19:6.

In the book of Revelation, the same phrase is again applied twice to those redeemed by faith in Jesus Christ. In Revelation 1:5-6, we read: *"Unto him* [Christ] *that loved us, and washed us from our sins in his own blood, and hath made us kings and priests unto God and his Father."* And again in Revelation 5:9-10: *"*[Thou] *hast redeemed us to God by thy blood....And hast made us unto our God kings and priests."* In all, God's purpose to make His redeemed people *"a kingdom of priests"* is stated four times in Scripture—once in the Old Testament and three times in the New Testament. In all three instances in the New Testament, God's purpose is presented, not as something yet to take place in the future, but as a fact already accomplished for us as Christians through our position in Christ.

We Rule by Prayer

In Psalm 110:1-4, David paints a picture of Christ reigning as King and Priest together with His believing people. Every detail of the scene is significant and merits our careful attention. The inspired language and imagery David uses must be interpreted by reference to other related passages of Scripture.

In the first verse, we have the revelation of Christ as King, enthroned at the Father's right hand: *"The Lord said unto my Lord, Sit thou at my right hand, until I make thine enemies thy footstool."* No other verse of the Old Testament is quoted more often in the New Testament than this. In three of the gospels, Jesus quotes the words of David and applies them to Himself (Matthew 22:44; Mark 12:36; Luke 20:42-43). They are likewise applied to Jesus by Peter in his sermon on the day of Pentecost (Acts 2:34-35). The truth of Christ's kingship is similarly presented by David in Psalm 2:6, where the Father declares: *"Yet have I set my king upon my holy hill of Zion."*

In verse 4 of Psalm 110, David's picture is completed by the revelation of Christ as Priest: *"The Lord hath sworn, and will not repent, Thou art a priest for ever after the order of Melchizedek."* The whole teaching of the Epistle to the Hebrews concerning Christ's high priesthood is based on this verse of Psalm 110. The writer of Hebrews stresses that in Melchizedek there was the union of the two functions of kingship and priesthood. Melchizedek was *"priest of the most high God."* In addition, he was, by the very meaning of his name, *"King of righteousness, and after that also King of Salem, which is, King of Peace"* (Hebrews 7:1-2).

Such is the double ministry that Christ now exercises at the Father's right hand. As King, He rules. As Priest, He intercedes: *"He ever liveth to make intercession"* (Hebrews 7:25).

Verse two describes the way in which Christ's kingly authority is exercised: *"The Lord shall send the rod of thy strength out of Zion: rule thou in the midst of thine enemies."* This is the situation in the world today. The enemies of Christ have not been finally subdued, but are still actively at work, opposing

His rule and His kingdom. However, Christ has been exalted and given authority over them all. Thus He rules now *"in the midst of His enemies."*

David speaks of *"the rod of thy strength"* (Psalm 110:2). It is by this that Christ rules. The *"rod"* in Scripture is the mark of a ruler's authority. When Moses stretched out his rod, the plagues of God came upon Egypt and later the waters of the Red Sea parted before Israel (Exodus chapters 7-14). As high priest and head over the tribe of Levi, Aaron had a rod on which his name was inscribed. (See Numbers 17:3.) The same applies to Christ. His authority is made effective by the use of His name.

In the scene painted by David, the rod is not stretched forth by Christ's own hand, but is sent forth *"out of Zion."* All through Scripture, Zion denotes the place of assembly of God's people. Speaking to Christians, the writer of Hebrews says: *"But ye are come unto mount Sion...to the general assembly and church of the firstborn which are* [enrolled] *in heaven"* (Hebrews 12:22-23). By right of our heavenly citizenship, we take our place in this assembly that is gathered in Zion.

Here we play our part in the double ministry of Christ. As kings, we rule with Him. As priests, we share His ministry of prayer and intercession. We must never seek to separate these two functions from each other. If we would rule as kings, we must serve as priests. The practice of our priestly ministry is the key to the exercise of our kingly authority. It is through prayer and intercession that we administer the authority that is ours in the name of Jesus.

How wonderfully David's picture illustrates the church's ministry of prayer! In the world, the forces of evil are rampant on every hand, rejecting the authority of Christ and opposing the work of His kingdom. But *"in the midst,"* the Christians assemble in divine order as kings and priests. Out of their assembly the rod of Christ's authority, exercised in His name, is *"sent forth"* through their prayers. In every direction that the rod is extended, the forces of evil are compelled to yield, and Christ in turn is exalted and His kingdom advanced.

All Christians look forward to the day when Christ's enemies shall have been finally and completely subdued, and He shall be openly manifested and universally acknowledged as King. The Bible promises that that day will come. But we must not let the promised glory of the future blind us to the reality of Christ's present position at God's right hand. **Christ rules even now** *"in the midst of His enemies,"* **and we rule with Him**. It is our responsibility to exercise the authority that is ours through His name, and in face of all the forces of evil to demonstrate that Christ is already *"King of kings and Lord of lords."*

3

Praying for Our Government

C hrist is *"King of kings and Lord of lords."*
His is the Ruler of earth's rulers and the
Governor over earth's governments. His authority over all earthly governments is made
available in His name to the church—the assembly of His believing people. As Moses
stretched forth his rod on God's behalf over
Egypt, so the church by its prayers stretches
forth Christ's authority over the nations and
their rulers.

Good Government Is God's Will

In his first letter to Timothy, Paul in-
structs him in the proper administration and

order of the local church, which he calls God's house. (See 1 Timothy 3:14-15.) Paul also gives directions for the church's ministry of prayer:

> *I exhort therefore, that, first of all, suppli-*
> *cations, prayers, intercessions, and giving*
> *of thanks, be made for all men;*
> *For kings, and all that are in authority;*
> *that we may lead a quiet and peaceable life*
> *in all godliness and honesty.*
> *For this is good and acceptable in the sight*
> *of God our Savior;*
> *Who will have all men to be saved, and to*
> *come unto the knowledge of the truth.*
> *(1 Timothy 2:1-4)*

"*First of all,*" Paul calls for "*supplications, prayers, intercession, and giving of thanks.*" If we were to choose one term to cover all four activities, it would be prayer. The first duty of Christians meeting in fellowship is prayer. It is also their primary outreach.

In the second verse, Paul says that prayer is to be offered "*for all men.*" This agrees with the prophecy of Isaiah 56:7 where God says, "*mine house shall be called an house of prayer for all people.*" God is concerned with "*all men*" and "*all people.*" He expects His people to share His concerns. Contrast this with the narrow, self-centered prayers of many professing Christians! Someone offered the following as a parody of the average church member's prayer: "God bless me, my wife, my son John and his wife. Us four. No more. Amen!"

After *"all men,"* the first specific topic for prayer is *"kings, and all that are in authority."* In countries such as the United States, which have no monarchy, the word *"kings"* does not apply. In any case, whether there be a monarchy or not, the phrase, *"all that are in authority,"* indicates all those who are responsible for governing the nation. This may be summed up in the single word, the government.

Thus, the first specific topic of prayer ordained by God for His people meeting in fellowship is the government. Extensive experience has convinced me that the vast majority of professing Christians never give any serious consideration to this topic in prayer. Not merely do they not pray for the government *"first,"* they scarcely pray for it at all! They pray regularly for groups such as the sick, the shut-ins, preachers, missionaries, evangelists, the unconverted—anything and everybody but the one group that God puts first—the government. It is no exaggeration to say that many who claim to be committed Christians never pray seriously for the government of their nation as much as once a week!

When praying for the government, what specific petition are we exhorted to make? In the second verse, Paul answers: *"that we may lead a quiet and peaceable life in all godliness and honesty."* Does the kind of government we live under affect the way we live? Obviously it does. Therefore, if we desire a good way of life, logic and self-interest alike indicate that we should pray for our government.

This was brought home to me in a new way when I applied for United States citizenship. Like all who make application, I was required to study in outline the basic principles and purposes of the American Constitution. As I meditated on these, I asked myself, "What was the real objective of those who originally drafted that Constitution?" I concluded that their objective could be summed up with complete accuracy in the words of Paul: *"that we may lead a quiet and peaceable life in all godliness and honesty."* The authors of the Constitution had as their objective a state in which every citizen would be free to pursue his own legitimate interests without interference from other citizens or the government, but with the protection of the government and its officers. Judged by the language which they used, most —if not all—of those who drafted the Constitution viewed such a state as being possible only under the sovereign protection and favor of Almighty God. Christian citizens of the United States should forever be thankful that the basic charter of their nation agrees so exactly with the purposes and principles of government ordained by Scripture.

Continuing in First Timothy 2, Paul says in verse 3, *"For this is good and acceptable in the sight of God our Savior."* The pronoun this refers back to the topic of verse 2, which we have summarized as "good government." If we replace the pronoun this by the phrase to which it refers, we arrive at the following statement: "Good government is good and acceptable in the sight of God." More simply still, "Good government is the will of God."

Here is a statement with the most far-reaching consequences. Do we really believe it? To judge by the words and actions of many Christians, they have little or no expectation of good government. They are more or less resigned to the fact that the government will be inefficient, wasteful, arbitrary, corrupt, unjust. For my part I have studied this question long and carefully in the light of logic and of Scripture, and I have come to a deep conviction concerning God's will in this area: **The will of God is good government**.

Why God Desires Good Government

Moving on to verse 4, we find that Paul states the reason why good government is the will of God: God desires *"all men to be saved, and to come unto the knowledge of the truth."* God desires the salvation of all men so intensely that He made it possible by the supreme sacrifice of history, the atoning death of Jesus Christ on the cross. Through faith in Christ's atonement, salvation has been made available to all men. However, for men *"to be saved,"* they must first *"come to the knowledge of the truth"* concerning Christ's atonement. This is possible only if they have the Gospel preached to them.

Paul presents this issue very plainly in Romans 10:13-14: *"For whosoever shall call upon the name of the Lord shall be saved. How then shall they call on him in whom they have not believed? and how shall they believe in him of whom they have not heard? and how shall they hear without a preacher?"* Unless the Gospel is preached to them, men cannot avail themselves of the salvation purchased for them by Christ's atonement.

We may sum up the logic of this very simply. God desires *"all men to be saved."* For this it is necessary for them to *"come to the knowledge of the truth."* *"Knowledge of the truth"* comes only through the preaching of the Gospel. Therefore God desires the Gospel to be preached to all men.

It remains only to trace the connection between good government and the preaching of the Gospel. We may do this by asking ourselves one simple question: Which kind of government makes it easier to preach the Gospel? Good government? Or bad government? To obtain an answer to this question, we may briefly contrast the effects of good and bad government, in so far as they relate to the preaching of the Gospel.

On the one hand, good government maintains law and order, it keeps communications open, it preserves civil liberty, it protects freedom of speech and freedom of assembly. (It is noteworthy that nearly all these points are specifically covered by the Constitution of the United States.) In short, good government, without becoming involved in religious controversy, provides a climate in which the Gospel can be preached effectively.

On the other hand, bad government allows the breakdown of law and order, permits unsafe travel conditions and poor communications, and imposes unjust and arbitrary restrictions. In all these ways, although in varying degrees, bad government hinders the effective preaching of the truth. At its worst, bad government either restricts or totally suppresses the universal right of all men to believe in God and to express their faith by public worship and proclamation. In one degree or another, we see these conditions in countries under communist rule today.

Our conclusion therefore is that good government facilitates the preaching of the Gospel, while bad government hinders it. For this reason, good government is the will of God.

We are now in a position to present the teaching of 1 Timothy 2:1-4 in a series of simple logical steps:

1. The first ministry and outreach of believers as we meet together in regular fellowship is prayer.
2. The first specific topic for prayer is the government.
3. We are to pray for good government.
4. God desires all men to have the truth of the Gospel preached to them.
5. Good government facilitates the preaching of the Gospel, while bad government hinders it.
6. Therefore, **good government is the will of God**.

Praying with the Knowledge of God's Will

The final sentence of the above summary has the most far-reaching consequences for our prayers. In all effective praying the decisive issue is the knowledge of God's will. If we know that what we are praying for is according to God's will, then we have faith to claim it. But if we are not sure of God's will, our prayers are wavering and ineffective. In James 1:6-7, James warns us that such wavering prayers will not be answered: *"For he that wavereth is like a wave of the sea driven with the wind and tossed. For let not that man think that he shall receive anything of the Lord."*

On the other side, John describes the confidence that comes from the assurance of God's will: *"And this is the confidence that we have in him* [God], *that, if we ask anything according to his will, he heareth us: And if we know that he hear us, whatsoever we ask, we know that we have the petitions that we desired of him"* (1 John 5:14-15).

John's teaching in this passage revolves around the knowledge of God's will. Provided that we know we are praying in full accord with God's will, we may know that *"we have"* whatsoever we prayed for. The use of the present tense *"we have"* does not necessarily indicate an immediate manifestation of the thing that we prayed for, but it does indicate an immediate assurance that the thing is already granted to us by God. Thereafter the amount of time taken for its actual manifestation cannot affect this initial assurance.

This agrees with the teaching of Mark 11:24: *"Therefore I say unto you, What things soever ye desire, when ye pray, believe that ye receive them* [more properly, believe that you already received them], *and ye shall have them."* Receiving comes at the very moment of praying. After that, the actual manifestation of that which we have received follows at the appropriate time.

With this preliminary explanation, it is now possible to apply to 1 John 5:14-15 the same kind of logical analysis that we have already applied to 1 Timothy 2:1-4. John's teaching in these verses may be summed up as follows:

1. If we know that we are praying for anything according to God's will, we know that He hears us.
2. If we know that God hears us, we know that we have the thing that we prayed for. (This does not necessarily indicate immediate fulfillment.)

To comprehend fully what we can accomplish by praying for our government, we need to combine the teaching of John with that of Paul. The result is as follows:

1. If we pray for anything knowing that it is according to God's will, we have the assurance that the thing is granted to us.
2. Good government is according to God's will.
3. If we know this and pray for good government, we have the assurance that good government is granted to us.

Why, then, do the majority of Christians have no assurance of good government? There can only be two reasons: either they do not pray at all for good government; or they pray for good government, but without the knowledge that it is God's will.

These conclusions drawn from Scripture have been confirmed by my personal observations. The great majority of Christians never pray seriously for good government at all. Of the few who do pray for good government, hardly any do so with the scriptural conviction that it is really God's will. Whichever of these explanations may apply in any given situation, the conclusion remains the same: **God has made it possible for Christians by their prayers to insure good government**. Christians who fail to exercise this God-given authority are gravely delinquent—both toward God and toward their countries.

Having been raised in Britain, I am frequently shocked by the way in which Americans habitually speak about the officers of their government. I do not know of any European nation—either outside or inside the Iron Curtain—where people would permit themselves to speak about their rulers with the disrespect and cynicism regularly heard in America. The irony of this is that, in an elective democracy, those who continually criticize their rulers are, in effect, criticizing themselves, since it is within their power by the processes of election to change those rulers and to replace them by others. This applies with double force to Christians in such a democracy, who, in addition to the normal political machinery, have also available to them the God-given power of prayer by which to bring about the changes which they believe desirable, either in the personnel or in the policy of the government.

The truth is that Christians are not held responsible by God to criticize their government, but they are held responsible to pray for it. **So long as they fail to pray, Christians have no right to criticize.** In fact, most political leaders and administrators are more faithful in the discharge of their secular duties than Christians are in the discharge of their spiritual duties. Furthermore, if Christians would seriously begin to intercede, they would soon find less to criticize.

I am persuaded that the root of the problem with most Christians is not lack of will, but lack of knowledge. Let this fact first be clearly established: Good government is God's will. This will provide both the faith and the incentive that Christians need to pray effectively for their government.

4

Rulers Are God's Agents

In politics, as in many other fields of activity, men continually strive for promotion. Yet few seriously ask the question: Where does promotion come from? What power is it that exalts men to positions of authority, or removes them from such positions?

Promotion Comes from God

In Psalm 75, the Bible deals very directly with this question:

I said unto the fools, Deal not foolishly:
and to the wicked, Lift not up the horn:
Lift not up your horn on high: speak not
with a stiff neck.

> *For promotion cometh neither from the
> east, nor from the west, nor from the south.
> But God is the judge: he putteth down one,
> and setteth up another.* (Psalm 75:4-7)

The psalmist begins by warning men
against their own self-confidence and arrogance. To *"lift up the horn"* suggests the desire
for personal aggrandizement. To *"speak with a
stiff neck"* suggest boastful self-assertiveness.
These are not the ways to promotion. Indeed,
promotion does not come from the earthly
level. We may interpret the three directions
east, west, and south as representing the various sources to which men are prone to look for
political aggrandizement, such as wealth, education, social position, influential connections,
and military power. For men to seek their own
exaltation from sources such as these is to
"deal foolishly." Promotion comes from God.
He is the one who both raises men up and puts
them down.

The record of the forty-one men who have
hitherto held office as President of the United
States is a remarkable confirmation that the
source of political power is outside the men
who themselves exercise it. This is well illustrated by a passage from the writings of the
late President John F. Kennedy:

This insight into the nature of governing affirms the lesson of our history that there is no program of vocational training for the presidency; no specific area of knowledge that is peculiarly relevant. Nor are qualities of great leadership drawn from any particular section of the country or section of society. Nine of our Presidents, among them some of the most brilliant in office, did not attend college; whereas Thomas Jefferson was one of the great scholars of the age and Woodrow Wilson the president of Princeton University. We have had Presidents who were lawyers and soldiers and teachers. One was an engineer and another a journalist. They have been drawn from the wealthiest and most distinguished families of the nation, and have come from poor and anonymous beginnings. Some, seemingly well endowed with great abilities and fine qualities, were unable to cope with the demands of the office, while others rose to a greatness far beyond any expectation.
(1962, Parade Publications, Inc. 733 Third Ave. New York, N.Y.)

If we turn back to the records of the kings of Israel, we find none who achieved a more spectacular rise to greatness than David. Beginning life as a poor shepherd boy, he ended his days in victory and honor as the ruler of a powerful empire. Unlike many other men who have achieved political greatness, David recognized the source of his success. In a prayer to God uttered near the end of his life, he ascribed his greatness solely to God: *"Both riches and honor come of thee, and thou reignest over all; and in thine hand is power and might; and in thine hand it is to make great, and to give strength unto all"* (1 Chronicles 29:12). Wise and happy is the ruler who acknowledges the true source of his power!

Daniel is another great character of the Bible who discovered the true source of political power. Challenged by King Nebuchadnezzar to reveal both the king's dream and its interpretation, he and his companions sought God in earnest prayer and received the answer by direct revelation (Daniel 2:17-19). In response, Daniel offered his prayer of gratitude and acknowledgment:

> *Blessed be the name of God for ever and ever: for wisdom and might are his:*
> *And he changeth the times and the seasons: he removeth kings, and setteth up kings: he giveth wisdom unto the wise, and knowledge to them that know understanding.*　　　　　　　*(Daniel 2:20-21)*

In the fourth chapter of Daniel, the prophet is again called upon to interpret a dream for

King Nebuchadnezzar. Concerning this dream Daniel tells the king:

> *This matter is by the decree of the watchers, and the demand by the word of the holy ones: to the intent that the living may know that the most High ruleth in the kingdom of men, and giveth it to whomsoever he will, and setteth up over it the basest of men.* (Daniel 4:17)

God wants men to acknowledge that He is the supreme ruler over all human affairs, and that earthly rulers are raised up by His decree. Not only so, but at times God actually raises up *"the basest of men"* as rulers.

How God Uses Human Rulers

Why should God raise up *"base men"* as rulers? The answer is supplied by the case of Nebuchadnezzar. God uses human rulers as instruments of judgment upon His own people. The Jewish nation had persistently offended against God by religious backsliding and social injustice. After many warnings, God set over them the cruel, idolatrous King Nebuchadnezzar. In a series of judgments that progressively increased in severity, Nebuchadnezzar first removed many of the Jews as captives to

Babylon and brought the nation under tribute. Finally, he destroyed the city of Jerusalem, together with the temple, and uprooted the whole nation out of their own land. Thus even in his baseness, Nebuchadnezzar was the instrument of God to bring judgment upon the backslidden and rebellious Jewish nation.

Yet Nebuchadnezzar is also a remarkable example of how God's grace and power can change an instrument of judgment into an instrument of mercy. When Daniel and his companions sought God in earnest prayer, God changed the heart of Nebuchadnezzar. On account of the special wisdom given by God to Daniel, Nebuchadnezzar raised him and his companions to positions of the highest power. Daniel's three companions became rulers of the province of Babylon, while Daniel himself became the prime minister of the entire Babylonian empire, with power second only to that of Nebuchadnezzar himself. This dramatic change, both in the personal attitude of Nebuchadnezzar and in the position of the Jews, was brought about by the prayers of Daniel and his companions.

The career of Daniel, like that of David, is in itself an example of God's ability to raise up a man from humble beginnings to a position of great political power. In his youth, Daniel had originally been taken to Babylon as a kind of political hostage. Yet within a short period he was elevated to the position of prime minister. Even after the fall of the Babylonian empire, we still find Daniel occupying a position of influence and authority in the succeeding Medo-Persian empire, under the rulership of Darius and Cyrus.

We are given a glimpse of Daniel's prayer life in Daniel chapter 6. The story indicates that his practice of regular prayer was well known in the court of Darius. Motivated by jealousy, Daniel's rivals seized upon this as a means to incriminate him. They persuaded Darius to sign a decree by which, for the next thirty days, prayer was not to be offered to any person except Darius. The penalty for disobeying this decree was death by being cast into the lions' den.

Daniel's response is recorded in verse 10: *"Now when Daniel knew that the writing was signed, he went into his house; and his windows being open in his chamber toward Jerusalem, he kneeled upon his knees three times a day, and prayed, and gave thanks before his God, as he did aforetime."*

What a standard Daniel sets for all who follow him in the ministry of intercession! What a pattern of dedication and persistence! His face was set toward Jerusalem. Three times every day he prayed for the restoration of the city and for the return of Israel from exile to its own land. His continuing intercession on behalf of his people was a personal commitment so solemn and so urgent, that not even the threat of death could deter him.

The outcome of Daniel's intercession is recorded in 2 Chronicles:

> *Now in the first year of Cyrus king of Persia, that the word of the Lord spoken by the mouth of Jeremiah might be accomplished, the Lord stirred up the spirit and Cyrus king of Persia, that he made a proclamation throughout all his kingdom, and put it also in writing, saying,*
>
> *Thus saith Cyrus king of Persia, All the kingdoms of the earth hath the Lord God of heaven given me; and he hath charged me to build him an house in Jerusalem which is in Judah. Who is there among you of all his people? The Lord his god be with him, and let him go up.*
>
> *(2 Chronicles 36:22-23)*

In this way God fulfilled the promises of Israel's restoration which He had previously given, both through Isaiah and through Jeremiah. The promise given through Isaiah is found in Isaiah 44:26-28, and that given through Jeremiah is found in Jeremiah 25:12.

Here indeed is a very clear example of God changing human governments in the interests of His own people. On the one hand, God brought judgment upon the king of Babylon and his people because they stood in the way of the return of the Jews to Jerusalem and the rebuilding of the temple. (The king of Babylon here referred to was a successor of Nebuchadnezzar.) On the other hand, God raised up in their place Cyrus and the Medo-Persian empire, and made them the instruments of mercy and restoration for the Jews and Jerusalem.

Behind these events that changed the course of world empires, there were **two unseen spiritual forces at work: the Word of God spoken through His prophets, and the intercessory prayer** of Daniel.

From these examples of God's dealings with the Jewish nation through the instrumentality of Nebuchadnezzar and Cyrus, certain important principles emerge:

1. God uses human rulers as instruments to fulfill His purposes in history, particularly as they relate to His own covenant people.
2. If God's people are disobedient and rebellious, God subjects them to cruel and evil rulers.

3. If through repentance and prayer God's people lay claim upon His mercy, He may bring about a change of government in one or other of two ways: either by removing an evil ruler and replacing him by a good one; or by changing the heart of a cruel ruler, so as to make him an instrument of mercy rather than of judgment.

"For Your Sakes"

These principles, derived from historical examples of the Old Testament, are confirmed by the teaching given to Christians in the New Testament. In 2 Corinthians 4:15, Paul says: *"For all things are for your sakes."* God's dealings with the whole world have one supreme objective: the fulfillment of His purposes for His own people, related to Him through faith in Jesus Christ. Over all the events of the last two thousand years of world history, God has inscribed one all-inclusive heading, addressed to His people: *"For your sakes."*

In Romans, Paul applies this principle specifically to those who hold the office of government:

> *Every person must submit to the supreme authority. There is no authority but by act*

*of God, and the existing authorities are in-
stituted by him; consequently anyone who
rebels against authority is resisting a divine institution, and those who so resist
have themselves to thank for the punishment they will receive. For government, a
terror to crime, has no terrors for good be-
havior. You wish to have no fear of the
authorities? Then continue to do right and
you will have their approval, for they are
God's agents working for your good. But if
you are doing wrong, then you will have
cause to fear them; it is not for nothing
that they hold the power of the sword, for
they are God's agents of punishment, for
retribution on the offender. That is why
you are obliged to submit. It is an obligation imposed not merely by fear of retribution but by conscience.*

(Romans 13:1-5 NEB)

Out of this passage, we may select three
statements that are particularly significant:
"There is no authority but by act of God."
"They are God's agents working for your
good," or alternatively, "They are God's agents
of punishment." Paul addresses these words
specifically to Christians. He states that government is established by an act of God. How
that government will affect Christians depends
upon the attitude and conduct of the Christians. If they are walking in obedience to the

will of God, then the government and its officers *"are God's agents working for their good."*
But if Christians are disobedient and not walking in the path of God's will, then the government and its officers become *"God's agents of punishment."* This may all be summed up in one brief sentence: **Christians get the kind of government they deserve**.

What if Christians find themselves under a government that is evil? It may be corrupt, inefficient, wasteful, or again it may be actively cruel and oppressive towards Christians. How are Christians to react? God's Word gives them no liberty either to complain or to disobey. It does, however, impose upon them a solemn obligation to pray for their government. If they will humble themselves before God and meet His conditions, He will then hear their prayers and will *"for their sakes"* bring about a change of government that will ensure the fulfillment of His purposes and the best interests of His people.

What God Requires in Those Who Rule

Since it is within the power of Christians to determine by their prayers the kind of government they are to live under, it is important that we know what kind of government to pray for. What are God's main requirements in one who governs? The answer to this question is given by the Holy Spirit through the lips of David in 2 Samuel:

> *The Spirit of the Lord spake by me, and*
> *his word was in my tongue.*
> *The God of Israel said, the Rock of Israel*
> *spoke to me, He that ruleth over men must*
> *be just, ruling in the fear of God.*
> *And he shall be as the light of the morn-*
> *ing, when the sun riseth, even morning*
> *without clouds; as the tender grass spring-*
> *ing out of the earth by clear shining after*
> *rain.* (2 Samuel 23:2-4)

Two simple requirements for a ruler are here stated: **He must be just, and he must rule in the fear of God**. No doubt there is a prophetic reference here to the kingdom of Christ, and these words will find their complete and final fulfillment only in Christ. Nevertheless, the general principle is firmly established and applied to every man who exercises government. God's two requirements are that he shall be just and God-fearing. Whenever such a man is raised up to rule, God promises that blessings will follow: *"He shall be as the light of the morning, when the sun riseth, even a morning without clouds; as the tender grass springing out of the earth by clear shining after rain."*

The simplicity of God's requirements cuts across most of the motives and the pressures with which we are familiar in contemporary politics. In the United States and in Britain alike, there is firmly established a system of two-party government. In the United States, the two parties are Democrats and Republicans. In Britain, there are the Labor and Conservative parties. The names are different in the two countries, but the basic attitudes are similar.

Unfortunately, Christians in both countries often allow themselves to be more influenced by party sentiments or affiliations than by divine requirements. God does not promise blessing to a government upon the condition that it carry a particular party label—whether that label be Republican or Democrat, Conservative or Labor. God promises blessing to a government whose officers fulfill two great basic moral requirements. He demands that they be **just** and **God-fearing**. Wherever possible, Christians who respect God's requirements should make it a principle not to vote for any man who is not just and God-fearing, no matter what party label he may wear. If Christians ignore God's requirements and vote for men who are morally unworthy, they are actually inviting God to make those men, if elected, agents of His judgment against the very people who voted them into office.

In the United States particularly, the proportion of committed Christians within the total community is large enough to permit them to exercise a powerful influence over the type of men put forward as candidates for office. This was originally pointed out early in the nineteenth century by the great evangelist Charles Finney. Christians of all political backgrounds should agree upon one basic principle: **to withhold their votes from any candidates who do not fulfill the moral requirements established by Scripture**. If this principle were clearly established and firmly adhered to, each of the major political parties would be under pressure to put forward as their candidates only such men as fulfilled these requirements. The result would be to raise the standards of political conduct and government throughout the whole nation.

In other countries, and under other systems of government, God's people are not always in a position to apply this kind of political pressure. Nevertheless, they are still responsible to pray for the rulers of their nation, and in this way to exercise a decisive influence upon the course of government.

5

Seeing History Shaped through Prayer

For me the power of prayer to shape history is no mere abstract theological formula. I have seen it demonstrated in my own experience on many occasions. In this chapter, I will relate four such occasions. To make them effective as illustrations, I have chosen situations in which different nations and different political factors were involved.

The War in North Africa

From 1941 to 1943, I served as a hospital attendant with the British forces in North Africa. I was part of a small medical unit that worked with two British armored divisions—the First Armored Division and the Seventh

Armored Division. It was this latter division that became celebrated as the "desert rats," with the emblem of the white jerboa.

At that time the morale of the British forces in the desert was very low. The basic problem was that the men did not have confidence in their officers. I myself am the son of an army officer, and many of the friends with whom I grew up were from the same background. I thus had some valid standards of judgment. As a group, the officers in the desert at that time were selfish, irresponsible, and undisciplined. Their main concern was not the well-being of the men, or even the effective prosecution of the war, but their own physical comfort.

I recall one officer who became sick with malaria and was evacuated to a base hospital in Cairo. For his transportation to Cairo, he required one four-berth ambulance for himself, and a one-and-a-half-ton truck to carry his equipment and personal belongings. At the time, we were continually being reminded that trucks and gasoline were in very short supply, and that every effort must be made to economize in the use of both. From Cairo, this officer was then evacuated to Britain (a procedure that certainly was not necessitated by a mere bout of malaria). Some months later, we heard him on a radio broadcast relayed from Britain.

He was giving a very vivid account of the hardships of campaigning in the desert!

At that period our greatest hardship was the shortage of water. Supplies were very strictly rationed. Our military water bottles were filled every other day. This was all the water that we were allowed for every purpose—washing, shaving, drinking, cooking, etc. Yet the officers in their mess each evening regularly consumed more water with their whiskey than was allotted to the other ranks for all purposes combined.

The result of all this was the longest retreat in the history of the British army—about seven hundred miles in all—from a place in Tripoli called El Agheila to El Alamein, about fifty miles west of Cairo. Here the British forces dug in for one final stand. If El Alamein should fall, the way would be open for the Axis powers to gain control of Egypt, to cut the Suez Canal, and to move over into Palestine. The Jewish community there would then be subjected to the same treatment that was already being meted out to the Jews in every area of Europe that had come under Nazi control.

About eighteen months previously, in a military barrack room in Britain, I had received a very dramatic and powerful revelation of Christ. I thus knew in my own

experience the reality of God's power. In the
desert, I had no church or minister to offer me
fellowship or counsel. I was obliged to depend
upon the two great basic provisions of God for
every Christian: the Bible and the Holy Spirit.
I early came to see that, by New Testament
standards, fasting was a normal part of Christian discipline. During the whole period that I
was in the desert, I regularly set aside Wednesday of each week as a special day for fasting
and prayer.

During the long and demoralizing retreat
to the gates of Cairo, God laid on my heart a
burden of prayer, both for the British forces in
the desert and for the whole situation in the
Middle East. Yet I could not see how God could
bless leadership that was so unworthy and inefficient. I searched in my heart for some form
of prayer that I could pray with genuine faith
and that would cover the needs of the situation. After a while, it seemed that the Holy
Spirit gave me this prayer: "Lord, give us leaders such that it will be for Your glory to give us
victory through them."

I continued praying this prayer every day.
In due course, the British government decided
to relieve the commander of their forces in the
desert and to replace him with another man.
The man whom they chose was a general
named W. H. E. "Strafer" Gott. He was flown

to Cairo to take over command, but he was killed when his plane was shot down. At this critical juncture the British forces in this major theater of the war were left without a commander. Winston Churchill, then Prime Minister of Britain, proceeded to act largely on his own initiative. He appointed a more-or-less unknown officer, named B. L. Montgomery, who was hastily flown out from Britain.

Montgomery was the son of an evangelical Anglican bishop. He was a man who very definitely fulfilled God's two requirements in a leader of men. He was just and God-fearing. He was also a man of tremendous discipline. Within two months, he had instilled a totally new sense of discipline into his officers and had thus restored the confidence of the men in their leaders.

Then the main battle of El Alamein was fought. It was the first major allied victory in the entire war up to that time. The threat to Egypt, the Suez Canal and Palestine was finally thrown back, and the course of the war changed in favor of the Allies. Without a doubt, the battle of El Alamein was the turning point of the war in North Africa.

Two or three days after the battle, I found myself in the desert a few miles behind the advancing Allied forces. A small portable radio beside me on the tailboard of a military truck was relaying a news commentator's description of the scene at Montgomery's headquarters as he had witnessed it on the eve of the battle. He recalled how Montgomery publicly called his officers and men to prayer, saying, "Let us ask the Lord, mighty in battle, to give us the victory." As these words came through that portable radio, God spoke very clearly to my spirit, "That is the answer to your prayer."

How well this incident confirms the truth about promotion that is stated in Psalm 75:6-7. The British government chose Gott for their commander, but God set him aside and raised up Montgomery, the man of His own choosing. God did this to bring glory to His own name, and to answer a prayer which, by the Holy Spirit, He Himself had first inspired me to pray. By this intervention, God also preserved the Jews in Palestine from coming under the control of the Axis powers.

I believe that the prayer which God gave me at that time could well be applied to other situations, both military and political: "Lord, give us leaders such that it will be for Your glory to give us victory through them."

The Birth of the State of Israel

During 1947, the future of Palestine was brought before the General Assembly of the

United Nations. At that time the British still governed the country under a mandate that had been assigned to them by the League of Nations shortly after the end of World War I. On November 29, 1948, the United Nations voted to partition the country into two separate states, allotting a small area to an independent Jewish state and the rest of the country to the Arabs, with the city of Jerusalem under international control. The date set for the termination of the British mandate and the inception of the new political order in Palestine was May 14, 1948.

Almost immediately after the United Nations decision in favor of partition, the Arabs of Palestine, aided and abetted by' infiltrators from the surrounding Arab nations, embarked on an undeclared war against the Jewish communities in their midst. Several main areas of the country were virtually taken over by armed groups of Arabs, with little or no semblance of normal civil government. By the early part of 1948, the Jewish community inside Jerusalem already presented the appearance of a beleaguered city. They were almost totally cut off from supplies of food and other commodities, and were in a condition bordering on starvation.

On the date set for the inauguration of the new Jewish state, all the surrounding Arab nations simultaneously declared war on it. Something like 650,000 Jews, with the barest minimum of arms and equipment, and without any officially constituted military forces, found themselves confronted on every frontier by a hostile Arab world, fifty million strong, who boasted well-trained armies and abundant military supplies. The leaders of the Arab nations publicly declared their intention to annihilate the newborn Jewish state and to sweep the Jews into the sea.

At this period, my wife Lydia and I were living with our eight adopted daughters in the center of Jewish Jerusalem. We occupied a large house on the southeast corner of a main intersection between King George Avenue and a street leading eastward to the Jaffa Gate of the old city. Lydia had been living in or near Jerusalem for the previous twenty years. She had been an eyewitness to a long series of earlier conflicts in that area between the Arabs and the Jews. She recalled that invariably the Jews had been poorly armed and ill-prepared to resist attack. In this critical hour, it seemed that the odds against the Jews were immeasurably greater than on previous occasions, and the results of defeat too terrible to contemplate.

Together Lydia and I searched the Scriptures for words of encouragement or direction from God. Each day we became more and more convinced that we were living in the period of Israel's restoration, to which their prophets and leaders had looked forward over the long centuries of agony and exile. This was the time spoken of in Psalm 102:12-13: *"But thou, O Lord, shalt endure for ever....Thou shalt arise, and have mercy upon Zion: for the time to favor her, yea, the set time is come."*

We realized that we were seeing before our eyes the fulfillment of God's promise to Israel:

> *Fear not: for I am with thee: I will bring thy seed from the east, and gather thee from the west:*
> *I will say to the north, Give up; and to the south, Keep not back: bring my sons from far and my daughters from the ends of the earth.* (Isaiah 43:5-6)

These and other passages of Scripture convinced us that the restoration of the Jews to their land was the sovereign purpose of God being brought to fulfillment. If it was God's purpose to restore Israel, then it could not be His will for them to be driven out or destroyed. This gave us faith to pray for Israel's deliverance, based not on nationalistic prejudices, but on the scriptural revelation of God's will.

When Lydia and I were thus brought together by the Holy Spirit concerning God's will, our prayers fulfilled the condition stated in Matthew 18:19: *"Again I say unto you, That if two of you shall agree on earth touching any thing that they shall ask, it shall be done for them of my Father which is in heaven."* One day as we were praying together, I heard Lydia utter this short prayer: "Lord, paralyze the Arabs!"

When full-scale fighting broke out in Jerusalem, our house was less than a quarter of a mile from the front line, which ran more or less along the west wall of the old city. In the first six weeks of fighting, we counted approximately 150 windowpanes that had been broken by bullets. For most of this period, our whole family lived in a large laundry room in the basement.

Because of the strategic location of our house, our backyard was taken over by the Haganah—the volunteer Jewish defense force that later developed into the official Israeli army. An observation post under the command of a young man named Phinehas was located in the yard. Because of this, we became quite well acquainted with a number of the young Jewish people—both men and women—who manned the post.

Early in June of 1948, the United Nations succeeded in imposing a four-weeks' cease-fire, and there was a temporary lull in the fighting. One day during the cease-fire, some of our young Jewish friends were sitting in our living room, talking freely about their experiences in the initial period of fighting.

"There's something we can't understand," a young man said. "We go into an area where the Arabs are. They outnumber us ten to one and are much better armed than we are. Yet, at times, they seem powerless to do anything against us. It's as if they are paralyzed!"

Right there in our own living room, this young Jewish soldier repeated the very phrase that Lydia had uttered in prayer a few weeks previously! I have never since ceased to marvel at God's faithfulness. Not only did God literally answer Lydia's prayer to "paralyze the Arabs," but He also provided us with first-hand, objective testimony from a Jewish soldier in our own living room that this was what He had done! God's purpose to grant Israel continuing occupation of their land was, in this miraculous way, achieved with the loss of fewer lives than would otherwise have been the case.

It was the invading Arab armies, with all their superiority in arms and numbers, that were defeated and driven back. In the next

twenty years this initial victory of Israel was
consolidated by equally dramatic victories in
two succeeding wars. Today the state of Israel
has been firmly established and has achieved
amazing progress in almost every area of its
national life.

For Lydia and me all of this had greater
significance than the mere record of unusual
military or political achievements. Each time
we received some fresh news concerning Israel's continuing development and progress,
we said to ourselves with deep inner satisfaction: "Our prayers played a part in that."

The End of Stalin's Era

From 1949 to 1956, I was pastor of a congregation in London, England. I retained a
special interest in God's dealings with the Jewish people, which had first been kindled by my
experiences in Jerusalem at the time of the
birth of the state of Israel. Early in 1953, I received information from reliable sources that
Josef Stalin, who at that time ruled the Soviet
Union as an unchallenged dictator, was plan-
ning a systematic purge directed against the
Russian Jews.

As I meditated on this situation, the Lord
reminded me of Paul's exhortation to the gentile Christians concerning the Jews:

*For as ye in times past have not believed
God, yet have now obtained mercy through
their unbelief:
Even so have these also now not believed,
that through your mercy they also may obtain mercy.   (Romans 11:30-31)*

Somehow, I felt that God was laying at my
door the responsibility for the Jews in Russia. I
shared my feelings with the leaders of a few
small prayer groups in various parts of Britain,
who also had a special concern for the Jews.
Eventually, we decided to set aside one day for
special prayer and fasting on behalf of the
Russian Jews. I do not recall the exact date
chosen but I believe it was a Thursday. All the
members of our groups voluntarily committed
themselves to abstain from food that day and
to devote special time to prayer for God's intervention on behalf of the Jews in Russia. Our
own congregation met that evening for group
prayer devoted primarily to that topic.

There was no particularly dramatic spiritual manifestation in the meeting, no special
sense of being "blessed" or emotionally stirred.
But within two weeks from that day, the
course of history inside Russia was changed by
one decisive event: the death of Stalin. He was
seventy-three years old. No advance warning of
his sickness or impending death was given to

the Russian people. Up to the last moment, sixteen of Russia's most skilled doctors fought to save his life, but in vain. The cause of death was said to be a brain hemorrhage.

Let it be clearly stated that no member of any of our groups prayed for the death of Stalin. We simply committed the situation inside Russia to God, and trusted His wisdom for the answer that was needed. Nevertheless, I am convinced that God's answer came in the form of Stalin's death.

In Acts chapter 12, a somewhat similar answer to the prayers of the early church is recorded. King Herod had the apostle James, brother of John, executed. Then he proceeded to arrest Peter and hold him for execution immediately after the Passover. At this point, the church in Jerusalem applied themselves to earnest, persistent prayer on Peter's behalf. As a result, God intervened supernaturally through an angelic visitation, and Peter was delivered out of the prison. In this way, the prayers of the church for Peter were answered, but it still remained for God to deal with King Herod.

In the closing verses of the chapter, Luke gives a vivid picture of Herod, arrayed in his royal apparel, making a speech to the people of Tyre and Sidon. At the end of his oration, the people applauded, shouting, *"It is the voice of a god, and not of a man"* (Acts 12:22). Puffed up with conceit at his own achievements, Herod accepted the applause. However, the record concludes, *"Immediately an angel of the Lord struck him down because he did not give God the glory. And in fearful internal agony he died"* (12:23 PHILLIPS). The outworking of the power of prayer in human history can at times be swift and terrible.

It remains to point out the consequences of Stalin's death. The planned purge of Russian Jews was not carried out. Instead, a period of change in internal Russian policy was initiated, so significant and far-reaching that it later came to be known as the era of "destalinization." In due course, Stalin's successor and former associate, Khrushchev, denounced Stalin as a cruel and unjust persecutor of the Russian people. Later, Stalin's daughter, who had been raised under the teaching of atheistic communism, fled from her native land and sought refuge in the country which her father had persistently abused. She further professed her faith in a crucified Jew, whose followers her father had cruelly persecuted.

Kenya's Birth Pangs

From 1957 to 1961, Lydia and I served as educational missionaries in Kenya, East Africa.

I was the principal of a Teacher Training College in Western Kenya.

During this period, Kenya was still painfully struggling to recover from the bloody agonies of the Mau Mau movement, which had created bitter mistrust and hatred, not only between Africans and Europeans, but also among many of the various African tribes. At the same time, the country was being hastily prepared for the end of British rule and for national independence. This was eventually achieved in 1963.

In 1960, the Belgian Congo, which is to the west of Kenya, gained its independence. Without adequate preparation, the various different African groups inside the Congo were unable to meet the demands of self-government, and were plunged into a protracted series of bloody internal wars. Many of the European residents of the Congo fled eastward into Kenya, bringing with them gruesome pictures of the strife and chaos they had left behind them.

Against this background, the forecasts of the political experts for the future of Kenya were dark indeed. It was generally predicted that Kenya would follow the unhappy course of the Congo, but with problems made even more serious by the internal antagonisms that were the legacy of Mau Mau.

In August 1960, I was one of a number of missionaries ministering at a week-long convention for African young people held in western Kenya. There were about two hundred young Africans in attendance, most of whom were either teachers or students. A considerable number of these were either students or former students from the Teacher Training College of which I was the principal.

The convention ended on a Sunday. In the final service that evening, we witnessed a fulfillment of Joel's prophecy, quoted by Peter:

> *And it shall come to pass in the last days, saith God, I will pour out of my Spirit upon all flesh: and your sons and your daughters shall prophesy, and your young men shall see visions, and your old men shall dream dreams.* (Acts 2:17)

A missionary colleague from Canada brought the closing address, which was translated into Swahili by a young man named Wilson Mamboleo, who had recently graduated from our Teacher Training College. The first two hours of the service followed a normal pattern, but after the close of the missionary's address, the Holy Spirit moved with sovereign power and lifted the meeting onto a supernatural plane. For the next two hours, almost the whole group of more than two hundred people continued in spontaneous worship and prayer without any visible human leadership.

At a certain point, the conviction came to me that, as a group, we had touched God, and that His power was at our disposal. God spoke to my spirit, and said, "Do not let them make the same mistake that Pentecostals have so often made in the past, by squandering My power in spiritual self-indulgence. Tell them to pray for the future of Kenya."

I began to make my way to the platform, intending to deliver to the whole group the message which I felt God had given me. On the way, I passed Lydia, who was sitting beside the aisle. She put out her hand and stopped me.

"What do you want?" I asked her.

"Tell them to pray for Kenya," she said.

"That's just what I'm going up to the platform for," I replied. I realized that God had spoken to my wife at the same time that He had spoken to me, and I accepted this as confirmation of His direction.

Reaching the platform, I called the whole group to silence and presented God's challenge to them. "You are the future leaders of your people," I told them, "both in the field of education and also in the field of religion. The Bible places upon you, as Christians, the responsibility to pray for your country and its government. Your country is now facing the most critical period in its history. Let us unite together in praying for the future of Kenya."

Wilson Mamboleo was with me on the platform, translating my words into Swahili. When the time came to pray, he knelt down beside me. As I led in prayer, almost every person present joined me in praying out loud. The combined volume of voices rising in prayer reminded me of the passage in Revelation 19:6: *"And I heard as it were the voice of a great multitude, and as the voice of many waters, and as the voice of mighty thunderings."* The sound of prayer swelled to a crescendo, then suddenly ceased. It was as if some invisible conductor had brought down his baton.

After a few moments of silence, Wilson stood up and spoke to the congregation. "I want to tell you what the Lord showed me while we were praying," he said. I realized that God had given him a vision as he knelt beside me in prayer.

Wilson then related the vision he had seen, first in English and then in Swahili. "I saw a red horse approaching Kenya from the east," he said. "It was very fierce, and there was a very black man riding on it. Behind it were several other horses, also red and fierce. While we were praying, I saw all the horses turn around and move away toward the north."

Wilson paused for a moment, and then continued, "I asked God to tell me the meaning of what I had seen, and this is what He told me: 'Only the supernatural power of the prayer of my people can turn away the troubles that are coming upon Kenya!'"

For many days after that, I continued to meditate on what Wilson had told us. I realized that Wilson's vision was in some ways similar to one recorded in Zechariah 1:7-11. I asked Wilson whether he was familiar with this passage of Zechariah, and he replied that he was not. I gradually concluded that by this vision God had granted us an assurance that He had heard our prayers for Kenya, and that He would intervene in some definite way on behalf of the country. Subsequent events in Kenya's history have confirmed that this was so.

During the period of British rule, Kenya was one of three states that made up British East Africa. The other two states were Uganda to the west and Tanganyika to the south. (Tanganyika was later renamed Tanzania.) Kenya eventually achieved her independence on December 12, 1963. The other two states had already achieved independence somewhat earlier. Immediately after independence was declared, a national government was duly elected in Kenya, with Jomo Kenyatta as the nation's first president.

In January 1964, there was an exact outworking in Kenya's history of the vision which
Wilson had seen. A bloody revolution broke out
in Zanzibar, off Kenya's east coast. This was
led by an African from Uganda who had been
trained in revolutionary tactics under Castro
in Cuba. The revolution succeeded in over-
throwing the Sultan of Zanzibar.

In the same month, a revolutionary movement gripped the national army of Tanzania.
Its influence also spread to the army of Kenya.
The aim was to overthrow the elected government in Kenya and to replace it by a military
dictatorship under communist control.

At this critical point, Kenya's new president, Jomo Kenyatta, acted with wisdom and
firmness. Enlisting the help of the British
army, he suppressed the revolutionary movement in the Kenyan army and restored law
and order throughout the country. Thus, the
authority of Kenya's duly-elected government
was preserved, and the communist attempt at
a military take-over was completely foiled.

In Wilson's vision, the red horses that
turned away from Kenya moved towards the
north. Northward along the African coast from
Kenya lies Somalia. The kind of communist
military coup that failed in Kenya was successful in Somalia. Someone later described Somalia as "a communist military camp."

The other countries bordering on Kenya have likewise experienced serious political problems. To the south, in Tanzania, strong communist influence has brought about various limitations of political freedom. To the west, in Uganda, there has been a history of unstable governments and internal tribal clashes, with a very determined effort by the Moslems to gain control of the country and to make Islam the official religion of the nation. Yet in the midst of all this, Kenya has succeeded in combining order and progress with a high degree of political and religious liberty to a remarkable extent.

The attitude of Kenya's government toward Christianity has been consistently friendly and cooperative. Although President Kenyatta does not himself profess to be a Christian, he has officially invited the various Christian bodies in Kenya to teach the message of Christianity in every government school in the country. In many ways, Kenya has become a strategically located center from which trained national Christians are able to move out with the gospel message to all the surrounding countries.

Sometimes God uses unexpected means of getting information to us. In October 1966, I was in the office of a travel agency in Copenhagen, making arrangements for a flight to

London. While I was waiting for my ticket to be prepared, I picked up an English edition of the London Times. There was a special sixteen-page supplement which dealt exclusively with Kenya. In essence, the theme of this supplement was that Kenya had proved to be one of the most stable and successful of nearly fifty new nations that had emerged on the continent of Africa since the end of World War II. As I turned each page of the supplement, I seemed to hear the inaudible voice of God within my spirit, saying, "This is what I can do when Christians pray with faith for the government of their nation."

When I decided to record God's dealings with Kenya, I wrote to Wilson Mamboleo in Nairobi. I outlined my recollection of the vision which God had given him in 1960, and asked him to indicate any ways in which I could make my account more accurate. I also asked him if he had any comments to make on the then present situation in Kenya. The following are some extracts from his reply, dated June 30, 1972:

> Thank you for your letter. It is the Spirit of the living God who has guided you to ask me to write these things....
> It is so wonderful how the Lord has worked. I and another brother who loves

to pray have been uplifting you before the Lord in prayer and while we were doing so, I received your letter...

Concerning my vision of 1960, I feel you have grasped it well, so there wouldn't be any need for an addition...

At this time Kenya is leading a peaceful life. Economic development is steadily growing. Foreign investment is in a healthy structure. Business among the African people is booming in every town in the country. The success which is being achieved in Kenya is because of the stability of the present government led by His Excellency the President, "Mzee" Jomo Kenyatta.

I can say that God chose this man to lead our nation at such a time as this, and I, as well as many other faithful Christians in the country, do pray for him, that God may grant him wisdom.

Many people in the country do not have an answer who would be a successor to President Kenyatta, when his days on earth are over. In the eyes of men, there is no man of his caliber who will have such a commanding leadership, accepted by all his countrymen, as Kenyatta. However, I do believe, and this is what I tell those I meet, that "God will provide" a man—but only as a result of persistent prayer of the saints...

We thank God that Kenya enjoys more freedom to worship God in the way a person is led, than the other neighboring states. In Tanzania, religion—and especially Christianity—is being suppressed. Open-air evangelistic meetings are not allowed unless one has a valid permit from the authorities....In Uganda, the military government led by General Amin, a Moslem, is urging all religious bodies to become ecumenical. Recently General Amin himself made a mixture of worship—Moslem prayers were conducted in a Christian church, when the General himself attended the prayers....

The military government of Somalia is a socialist type of government. Somalia has close ties with the communist countries of the East—the Soviet Union and Red China. Large amounts of financial and material aids are given to Somalia, just as Tanzania receives its aid from China (including military training and supplies of Chinese MIG fighters)....

Over these past years, the history of Kenya and the surrounding nations has demonstrated the exact outworking of the vision which God gave to Wilson in 1960. The intervention of God on behalf of Kenya came through a group of Christians who united together to pray, in accordance with Scripture, for the government and the destiny of their nation.

As you ponder on this record of God's faithfulness, call to mind the words with which Wilson's vision closed: "Only the supernatural power of the prayer of my people can turn away the troubles that are coming upon Kenya."

Is there not good reason to believe that these words apply just as much to your country and to mine?

6

Fasting Intensifies Prayer

In the preceding chapter, various incidental references were made to the practice of fasting. It is now time to examine more systematically the teaching of Scripture on this subject. It will help to begin with a simple definition. We understand fasting to be the practice of deliberately abstaining from food for spiritual purposes. If abstinence from water (or other fluids) is also included, this is normally indicated by the context.

Christ's Teaching and Example

The best starting point for a study of the Christian discipline of fasting is to be found in the Sermon on the Mount. In Matthew 6:1-18 Christ gives instructions to His disciples on three related duties: giving alms, praying, and fasting. In each case, He places His main emphasis upon the motive and warns against religious ostentation for the sake of impressing men. With this qualification, He assumes that all His disciples will practice all three of these duties. This is indicated by the language which He uses concerning each.

In the second verse, He says, **"When** *thou doest alms...."* In verse six, He says, **"When** *thou* [singular] *prayest..."* (individually); and in the seventh verse, **"When** *ye* [plural] *pray..."* (collectively). In verse 16 He says, **"When** *ye* [plural] *fast..."* (collectively); and in verse 17, **"When** *thou* [singular] *fastest..."* (individually). In no case does Christ say *if*, but always *when*. The inference is clear. Christ expects that all His disciples will regularly practice all three of these duties. In particular, the parallel between prayer and fasting is exact. If Christ expects His disciples to pray regularly, then by the same token He expects them also to fast regularly.

Fasting was an accepted part of religious duty among the Jewish people in Christ's day. They had practiced it continuously from the time of Moses onward. Both the Pharisees and the disciples of John the Baptist fasted regularly. The people were surprised that they did not see the disciples of Jesus doing the same, and they asked Him the reason. Their question, and Christ's answer, are recorded in Mark:

> *And the disciples of John and of the Pharisees used to fast: and they come and say unto him, Why do the disciples of John and of the Pharisees fast, but thy disciples fast not?*
> *And Jesus said unto them, Can the children of the bridechamber fast, while the bridegroom is with them? As long as they have the bridegroom with them they cannot fast.*
> *But the days will come, when the bridegroom shall be taken from them and then shall they fast in those days.*
>
> *(Mark 2:18-20)*

This answer of Jesus is given in the form of a simple parable. It is important to interpret the parable correctly. The bridegroom, as always in the New Testament, is Christ Himself. The children of the bridechamber are the disciples of Christ (about whom the question had been asked). The period while the bridegroom is with them corresponds to the days of Christ's ministry on earth, while He was physically present with His disciples. The period when the bridegroom shall be taken from them commenced when Christ ascended back to heaven, and will continue until He returns for His church. In the meanwhile, the church, as a bride, is awaiting the return of the bridegroom. This is the period in which we are now living, and concerning which Jesus says very definitely, *"And then shall they* [the disciples] *fast in those days."* In the days in which we now live, therefore, fasting is a mark of true Christian discipleship, ordained by Jesus Himself.

Fasting is endorsed not merely by the teaching of Jesus, but also by His own personal example. Immediately after being baptized in the Jordan by John the Baptist, Jesus was led by the Holy Spirit to spend forty days fasting in the wilderness. This is recorded in Luke:

> *And Jesus being full of the Holy* [Spirit] *returned from Jordan, and was led by the Spirit into the wilderness,*
> *Being forty days tempted of the devil, and in those days he did eat nothing: and when they were ended, he afterward hungered.*
> *(Luke 4:1-2)*

The record says that Jesus did not eat at all during these forty days, but it does not say that He did not drink. Also it says that *"He afterward hungered,"* but it does not say that He was thirsty. The probable inference is, therefore, that He abstained from food, but not from water. During this period of forty days, Jesus came into direct spiritual conflict with Satan.

There is a significant difference in the expressions used by Luke to describe Jesus before and after His fast. At the beginning, in Luke 4:1, we read: *"And Jesus, being full of the Holy Spirit, returned from Jordan."* At the end, in Luke 4:14, we read: *"And Jesus returned in the power of the Spirit into Galilee."*

When Jesus went into the wilderness, He was already **full of the Holy Spirit**. But when He came out again after fasting, He returned in the **power of the Spirit**. It would appear that the potential of the Holy Spirit's power, which Jesus received at the time of His baptism in Jordan, only came forth into full manifestation after He had completed His fast. **Fasting was the final phase of preparation through which He had to pass, before entering into His public ministry**.

The same spiritual laws that applied in Christ's own ministry apply also in the ministry of His disciples. In John 14:12, Jesus says, *"He that believeth on me, the works that I do shall he do also."* By these words, Jesus opens the way for His disciples to follow in the pattern of His own ministry. However, in John 13:16, Jesus also says, *"The servant is not greater than his lord; neither he that is sent greater than he that sent him."* This applies to the preparation for ministry. If fasting was a necessary part of Christ's own preparation, it must play a part also in the disciple's preparation.

The Practice of the Early Church

In this respect, Paul was a true disciple of Jesus. Fasting played a vital part in his ministry. Immediately after his first encounter with Christ on the Damascus road, Paul spent the next three days without food or drink (Acts 9:9). Thereafter, fasting was a regular part of his spiritual discipline. In 2 Corinthians 6:3-10, Paul lists various different ways in which he had proved himself a true minister of God. In verse 5, two of the ways which he lists are: *"in watchings, in fastings."* *Watching* signifies going without sleep; *fasting* signifies going without food. Both were practiced at times by Paul to make his ministry fully effective.

In 2 Corinthians 11:23-27, Paul returns to this theme. Speaking of other men who set themselves up as his rivals in the ministry, Paul says: *"Are they ministers of Christ?...I am more."* He then gives another long list of ways in which he had proved himself a true minister of Christ. In verse 27, he says: *"In weariness and painfulness, in watchings often, in hunger and thirst, in fastings often."* Here again Paul joins watching with fasting. The plural form, *"in fastings often,"* indicates that Paul devoted himself to frequent periods of fasting. Hunger and thirst refers to occasions when neither food nor drink was available. *Fastings* refers to occasions when food was available, but Paul deliberately abstained for spiritual reasons.

The New Testament Christians not only practiced fasting individually, as a part of their personal discipline, but also practiced it collectively, as a part of their corporate ministry to God. This is attested to by Luke's account in Acts:

> *Now there were in the church that was at Antioch certain prophets and teachers; as Barnabas, and Simeon that was called Niger, and Lucius of Cyrene, and Manaen, which had been brought up with Herod the tetrarch, and Saul.*
> *As these ministered to the Lord, and fasted, the Holy* [Spirit] *said, Separate me Barnabas and Saul for the work whereunto I have called them.*
> *And when they had fasted and prayed, and laid their hands on them, they sent them away.* (Acts 13:1-3)

In this local congregation in the city of
Antioch, five leading ministers—designated as
prophets and teachers—were praying and fasting together. This is described as ministering
to the Lord. The majority of Christian leaders
or congregations today know very little of this
aspect of ministry. Yet, in the divine order,
**ministry to the Lord comes before minis-
try to men**. Out of the ministry to the Lord,
the Holy Spirit brings forth the direction and
the power needed for effective ministry to men.

So it was at Antioch. As these five leaders
prayed and fasted together, the Holy Spirit
revealed that He had a special task for two of
them—Barnabas and Saul (later called Paul).
He said, *"Separate me Barnabas and Saul for
the work whereunto I have called them."* In this
way these two men were called out for a special
task.

However, they were not yet ready to undertake the task. They still required the im-
partation of the special grace and power that
were needed for the task that lay ahead. For
this purpose, all five men fasted and prayed
together the second time. Then, after the second period of fasting, the other leaders laid
their hands on Barnabas and Paul, and sent
them forth to fulfill their task.

Thus, it was through collective prayer and
fasting that Barnabas and Paul received, first,

the revelation of a special task, and second, the grace and power needed to fulfill that task. At the time they all prayed and fasted together, Barnabas and Paul—like the other three men—were recognized as prophets and teachers. But after being sent forth to their task, they were described as apostles (see Acts 14:4, 14). We may therefore say that the apostolic ministry of Barnabas and Paul was born out of collective prayer and fasting by five leaders of the church at Antioch.

In due course, this practice of collective prayer and fasting was transmitted by Barnabas and Paul to the congregations of new disciples which were established in various cities as a result of their ministry. The actual establishment of each congregation was accomplished through the appointment of their own local elders. This is described in Acts:

> *And...they returned again to Lystra, and to*
> *Iconium, and Antioch,*
> *Confirming the souls of the disciples, and*
> *exhorting them to continue in the faith....*
> *And when they had ordained them elders*
> *in every church, and had prayed with*
> *fasting, they commended them to the Lord,*
> *on whom they believed.*   *(Acts 14:21-23)*

In Acts 14:22, these groups of believers in each city are referred to merely as disciples.

But in the next verse, the writer refers to them as churches. The transition from *"disciples"* to *"churches"* was accomplished by the appointment of the local leaders for each congregation, who were designated as *"elders."* In each case, when elders were appointed, *"they prayed with fasting."* It is therefore fair to say that the establishment of a local church in each city was accompanied by collective prayer and fasting.

Taken together, chapters 13 and 14 of the Book of Acts indicate that collective prayer and fasting played a vital role in the growth and development of the New Testament church. It was **through praying and fasting together that the early Christians received direction and power from the Holy Spirit for decisions or tasks of special importance**. In the examples which we have considered, these were: first, the appointment and sending forth of apostles; second, the appointment of elders and the establishment of local churches.

How Fasting Works

There are various ways in which fasting helps a Christian to receive direction and power from the Holy Spirit. In one sense, fasting is a form of mourning. Psychologically, no one welcomed the thought of mourning, just as, physically, no one welcomes the thought of fasting. Nevertheless, there are times when both mourning and fasting are beneficial. Mourning has its place among the beatitudes. In Matthew 5:4, Jesus says, *"Blessed are they that mourn: for they shall be comforted."* In Isaiah 61:3, the Lord promises special blessings to those who *"mourn in Zion."* He promises them *"beauty for ashes, the oil of joy for mourning, the garment of praise for the spirit of heaviness."*

Mourning in Zion is neither the self-centered remorse nor the hopeless grief of the unbeliever. Rather it is a response to the prompting of the Holy Spirit through which the believer shares in a small measure God's own grief over the sin and folly of humanity. When we consider our own failures and shortcomings as Christians, and when we look beyond ourselves at the misery and wickedness of the world, there is indeed cause for this kind of mourning. In 2 Corinthians 7:10, Paul contrasts the godly sorrow of the believer with the hopeless sorrow of the unbeliever: *"For godly sorrow worketh repentance to salvation not to be repented of: but the sorrow of the world worketh death."* Godly mourning of this kind is followed in due season by the oil of joy and the garment of praise.

Under the old covenant, God ordained for Israel one special day in each year in which they were to *"afflict their souls."* This was the Day of Atonement. In Leviticus 16:31, the Lord instructed Israel concerning this day: *"It shall be a sabbath of rest unto you, and ye shall afflict your souls by a statute for ever."* From the time of Moses onward, the Jews have interpreted this as a command to fast. In Acts 27:9, it is this annual Day of Atonement which is referred to as *"the fast."*

Nineteen centuries later, under its Hebrew name *Yom Kippur*, the Day of Atonement is still observed by Orthodox Jews all over the world as a day of fasting.

In two of his psalms, David also speaks of fasting in this way. In Psalm 35:13, he says, *"I humbled my soul with fasting."* The word here translated *"humble"* is the same that is translated *"afflict"* in the chapter on the Day of Atonement. Again in Psalm 69:10, David says, *"I wept, and chastened my soul with fasting."* We may combine the various expressions used and say that fasting, as here practiced, is a form of mourning and a means to humble oneself and to chasten oneself.

Fasting is also a means by which a believer brings his body into subjection. In 1 Corinthians 9:27, Paul says: *"But I keep under my body, and bring it into subjection: lest that by any means, when I have preached to others, I myself should be a castaway,"* Our bodies, with their physical organs and appetites, make wonderful servants, but terrible masters. Therefore it is necessary to keep them always in subjection. I once heard this well expressed by a fellow minister who said, "My stomach does not tell me when to eat, but I tell my stomach when to eat." Each time a Christian practices fasting for this purpose, he is serving notice on his body: "You are the servant, not the master."

In Galatians 5:17, Paul lays bare the direct opposition that exists between the Holy Spirit of God and the carnal nature of man: *"For the flesh lusteth against the Spirit, and the Spirit against the flesh: and these are contrary the one to the other."* Fasting deals with the two great barriers to the Holy Spirit that are erected by man's carnal nature. These are the stubborn self-will of the soul and the insistent, self-gratifying appetites of the body. **Rightly practiced, fasting brings both soul and body into subjection to the Holy Spirit**.

It is important to understand that fasting changes man, not God. The Holy Spirit, being God, is both omnipotent and unchanging. Fasting breaks down the barriers in man's carnal nature that stand in the way of the Holy Spirit's omnipotence. With these barriers removed, the Holy Spirit can work unhindered in His fullness through our prayers.

In Ephesians 3:20, Paul seeks to express the inexhaustible potential of prayer: *"Now unto him that is able to do exceeding abundantly above all that we ask or think, according to the power that worketh in us."* The power that works in and through our prayers is the Holy Spirit. By removing the carnal barriers, fasting makes a way for the Holy Spirit's omnipotence to work the *"exceeding abundantly above"* of God's promises.

There is indeed only one limit to God's omnipotence, and that is God's eternal righteousness. Fasting will never change the righteous standards of God. If something is outside the will of God, fasting will never put it inside the will of God. If it is wrong and sinful, it is still wrong and sinful, no matter how long a person may fast.

There is an example of this in 2 Samuel chapter 12. David committed adultery. Out of this a child was born. God said that part of the judgment was that the child would die. David fasted seven days, but the child still died. Fasting seven days did not change God's righteous judgment on David's sinful act. If a thing is wrong, fasting will not make it right. Nothing will do that.

Fasting is neither a gimmick nor a cureall. God does not deal in such things. God has made full provision for the total well-being of

His people in every area of their lives—spiritual, physical, and material. Fasting is one part of this total provision. Fasting is not a substitute for any other part of God's provision. Conversely, no other part of God's provision is a substitute for fasting.

In Colossians 4:12, we read that Epaphras prayed for his fellow believers that they might stand *"perfect and entire in all the will of God."* This sets a very high standard for all of us. One scriptural means provided for us to attain to this standard is fasting.

We may illustrate the relationship between fasting and the will of God by a simple diagram:

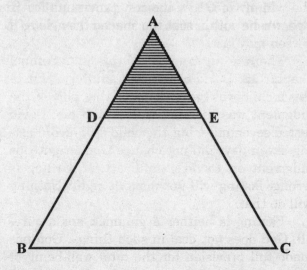

The whole triangle *ABC* represents the complete will of God for every believer. The truncated cone *DBCE* represents the area of God's will which may be appropriated by prayer without fasting. The smaller shaded triangle *ADE* represents the area of God's will that can be appropriated only by prayer and fasting combined.

If an objective is outside the area *ABC*, it is altogether outside God's will. There is no scriptural means by which we may obtain it. If an objective is in the area *DBCE*, we may obtain it by prayer without fasting. If an objective is in the area *ADE*, we may obtain it only by prayer and fasting combined.

Many of God's choicest provisions for His people lie within that top shaded triangle *ADE*.

7

Fasting Brings Deliverance and Victory

I f we turn to the historical records of the Old
Testament, we find a number of occasions
where collective fasting and prayer brought
forth dramatic and powerful intervention by
God. We will examine four such occasions.

Jehoshaphat Conquers without Fighting

Our first example is found in 2 Chronicles
20:1-30. Jehoshaphat, king of Judah, received
word that a very large army from the territo-
ries of Moab, Ammon, and Mount Seir was

invading his kingdom from the east. Realizing that he had no military resources with which to meet this challenge, Jehoshaphat turned to God for help. His first decisive act is described in verse 3: *"Jehoshaphat...proclaimed a fast throughout all Judah."* In this way God's people were called to unite in public, collective fasting and prayer for divine intervention. Verse 13 indicates that men, women, and children were all included.

From the initial call to fasting, events followed in swift succession, leading up to a dramatic climax. The first result is recorded in verse 4: *"And Judah gathered themselves together, to ask help of the Lord: even out of all the cities of Judah they came to seek the Lord."* Common danger had the effect of bringing all God's people together. The same emergency that threatened one community or one city threatened all alike. No doubt there were jealousies or rivalries between some of the cities represented. But in the face of the enemy invasion, these were set aside. God's people were called upon to protect their common inheritance rather than to promote their individual differences.

With the people of Judah thus assembled in one accord, Jehoshaphat led them in a prayer, reminding God of His covenant with Abraham and of His promises of mercy based on that covenant. Jehoshaphat's prayer received an immediate, supernatural response from God, which is described in verses 14 through 17. Through one of the Levites present, named Jahaziel, the Holy Spirit gave forth a powerful prophetic utterance, combining encouragement, assurance, and direction.

Jahaziel's prophetic utterance was received in turn with spontaneous worship and praise by Jehoshaphat and all the people. Thereafter, Jehoshaphat made provision for continuing, organized praise as he led his people forth to battle:

> *And Jehoshaphat bowed his head with his face to the ground: and all Judah and the inhabitants of Jerusalem fell before the Lord, worshipping the Lord.*
> *And the Levites...stood up to praise the Lord God of Israel with a loud voice on high.*
> *And when he* [Jehoshaphat] *had consulted with the people, he appointed singers unto the Lord, and that should praise the beauty of holiness, as they went out before the army, and to say, Praise the Lord; for his mercy endureth for ever.*
> *(2 Chronicles 20:18-19, 21)*

The outcome is described in verses 22 through 30. There was no need for God's people to use any kind of military weapon. The entire army of their enemies destroyed themselves, leaving not a single survivor. All that God's people needed to do was to spend three days gathering the spoils and then to return in triumph to Jerusalem, with their voices raised in loud thanksgiving and praise to God. Furthermore, the impact of this tremendous, supernatural victory was felt by all the surrounding nations. From then on, no other nation dared to contemplate hostilities against Jehoshaphat and his people.

Three practical lessons can be learned from Jehoshaphat's victory. All three apply with equal force to Christians in this age.

First of all, the anti-Christian forces that are at work in the world today are just as hostile and just as formidable as the army that threatened Judah in the days of Jehoshaphat. These forces are united in hatred and opposition toward all who truly love and serve the Lord Jesus Christ. They are not concerned about internal denominational distinctions among Christians. They are not disposed to spare the Baptists at the expense of the Methodists, nor the Catholics at the expense of the Pentecostals. Therefore, this is no time for Christians to emphasize sectarian or denominational issues that have in the past divided us. Rather, **it is time for all God's people** to follow the example of Judah **and to unite in fasting and prayer**.

Secondly, the story of Jehoshaphat demonstrates **the need for spiritual gifts**. It was the gift of prophecy that gave both encouragement and direction to Judah in their hour of crisis. The supernatural gifts of the Holy Spirit are still needed just as much by the church today. Nor does the Bible suggest that God ever intended to withdraw these gifts from the church.

In 1 Corinthians 1:7-8, Paul thanks God on behalf of the Corinthian believers, saying, *"So you are not lacking in any spiritual gift, as you wait for the revealing of our Lord Jesus Christ; who will sustain you to the end, guiltless in the day of our Lord Jesus Christ."* (RSV). Clearly, Paul both expected and desired that the spiritual gifts would continue to operate in the church right up to the return of Christ and the end of the age.

Likewise, Peter quotes the prophecy of Joel in Acts and applies it to our present age:

> *And it shall come to pass in the last days, saith God, I will pour out of my Spirit upon all flesh: and your sons and your daughters shall prophesy, and your young men shall see visions, and your old men shall dream dreams:*

> *And on my servants and on my handmaid-*
> *ens I will pour out in those days of my*
> *Spirit, and they shall prophesy.*
>
> *(Acts 2:17-18)*

These words of Joel, quoted by Peter, confirm those of Paul in 1 Corinthians. There is
no suggestion that the supernatural gifts of the
Holy Spirit are to be withdrawn from the
church, but rather that they are to be more
and more manifested, the nearer we come to
the end of the age.

The third lesson to be learned from the
story of Jehoshaphat is **the supremacy of
spiritual power over carnal power**. In 2
Corinthians 10:4, Paul says: *"For the weapons
of our warfare are not carnal, but mighty
through God."* There are two kinds of weapons: spiritual and carnal. Jehoshaphat's enemies relied on carnal weapons; Jehoshaphat
and his people used only spiritual weapons.
The outcome of the conflict demonstrates the
absolute supremacy of the spiritual over the
carnal.

What exactly were the **spiritual weapons** that Jehoshaphat used to such effect?
They may be briefly summarized as follows:
first, **collective fasting**; second, **united
prayer**; third, the **supernatural gifts of the
Holy Spirit**; fourth, **public worship and**

praise. These weapons, scripturally employed by Christians in this present day, will gain victories as powerful and dramatic as they gained for the people of Judah in the days of Jehoshaphat.

Ezra Obtains Safe Conduct from Heaven

For our second example of collective fasting and prayer, we will turn to Ezra:

> *Then I [Ezra] proclaimed a fast there, at the river of Ahava, that we might afflict ourselves before our God, to seek of him a right way for us, and for our little ones, and for all our substance.*
> *For I was ashamed to require of the king a band of soldiers and horsemen to help us against the enemy in the way: because we had spoken unto the king, saying,*
> *The hand of our God is upon all them for good that seek him....*
> *So we fasted and besought our God for this: and he was intreated of us.*
> *(Ezra 8:21-23)*

Ezra did something that you and I sometimes do. By testifying to the king, he put himself in a position where he had to live up to his own testimony. He had told the king: "We are the servants of the living God. Our God protects us and supplies all our needs." A little later the way opened for Ezra to lead a company of returning exiles back to Jerusalem. They had to make a long journey through country infested by savage tribes and by bandits. In addition to their wives and children, they had with them the sacred vessels of the temple, worth hundreds of thousands of dollars. What a prey for bandits!

The question arose: How were they to be protected on their way from Babylon to Jerusalem? Should Ezra go to the king and ask him for an escort of soldiers and horsemen? No doubt the king would have granted this request, but Ezra felt ashamed to make it because he had already testified to the king that their God, the true and living God, would protect those who served Him.

At this point, Ezra and the returning exiles made a vital decision: They would not rely on soldiers and horsemen for their protection, but on the supernatural power of God. There would not have been anything morally wrong in accepting an escort from the king, but it would have been depending on carnal means. Instead, by collective prayer and fasting, they committed themselves to seeking their help and protection solely frown the spiritual realm of God's power.

Ezra followed the same procedure as Jehoshaphat. As the leader of God's people, he *"proclaimed a fast."* The reason he gave for this was *"that we might afflict ourselves before our God, to seek of him a right way for us, and for our little ones, and for all our substance."* In our preceding chapter, we saw (both from the psalms of David and from the ordinances of the Day of Atonement) that fasting was recognized by the Jews, and approved by God, as a means whereby God's people might humble themselves before Him and acknowledge their total dependence upon Him. Ezra concludes by saying: *"So we fasted and besought our God for this: and he was intreated of us."*

The result of collective fasting and prayer for Ezra and his company was as decisive as it had been for Jehoshaphat and the people of Judah. The returning band of exiles completed their long and dangerous journey in perfect peace and safety. There was no opposition by bandits or savage tribes, no loss of persons or of property. Thus, the lesson demonstrated by Jehoshaphat was further confirmed by Ezra: **Victory in the spiritual realm is primary**. It is to be obtained by the employment of spiritual weapons. Thereafter, its outcome will be manifested in every area of the natural and material realm.

Esther Transforms Disaster into Triumph

Our third example of collective fasting and prayer is found in the fourth chapter of the Book of Esther. Here is described the greatest crisis that has ever confronted the Jewish people in their entire history up to the present time—greater even than the crisis under Adolph Hitler. Hitler had only one-third of all the Jews at his mercy. The Persian emperor had the entire Jewish nation. A decree went out that they were all to be annihilated on a certain day. The name of the man who was Satan's advocate against the Jews was Haman.

This story has given rise to the feast which the Jews call *Purim*. *Purim* means "lots." The feast is so called because Haman cast lots to determine the day that should be appointed for the destruction of the Jews. Casting lots was a form of divination. Haman was seeking guidance from occult powers. He relied on unseen spiritual forces to direct him in exterminating the Jews. This placed the whole conflict on the spiritual plane. It was not just flesh against flesh; it was spirit against spirit. Through Haman, Satan was actually challenging the power of God Himself. Had he succeeded in the destruction of the Jews, it would have been an everlasting reproach to the name of the Lord.

But when the decree for the destruction of the Jews went out, Esther and her maidens accepted the challenge. They understood that the conflict was on the spiritual plane, and their response was on the same plane. They agreed to fast three days, night and day, neither eating nor drinking. They arranged with Mordecai that he would gather together all the Jews in Shushan, the capital city, to unite with them in fasting for the same period. (Notice in Esther 2:19 that once again, in the hour of crisis, we find God's people were *"gathered together,"* just as in the days of Jehoshaphat.) Thus, all the Jews in Shushan, together with Esther and her maidens, fasted and prayed three days—seventy-two hours—without eating or drinking.

The outcome of their collective fasting and prayer is described in the succeeding chapters of the Book of Esther. We may summarize it briefly by saying that the whole policy of the Persian empire was completely changed, in favor of the Jews. Haman and his sons perished. The enemies of the Jews throughout the Persian empire suffered total defeat. Mordecai and Esther became the two most influential personalities in Persian politics. The Jews in every area experienced a unique measure of favor, peace, and prosperity. All this can be directly attributed to one cause: the collective fasting and prayer of God's people.

Nineveh Spared; Samaria Destroyed

We have taken our first three examples of collective fasting and prayer from the history of Israel. For our fourth and final example, we will turn to a gentile nation. The Book of Jonah records God's dealings with the city of Nineveh, the capital of Assyria, at that time the most powerful empire in the ancient world. The Bible pictures Nineveh as a cruel, violent, idolatrous city, ripe for divine judgment. God called Jonah to go and warn Nineveh that judgment was about to fall.

Jonah refused to go at first. He was a citizen of the northern kingdom of Israel. He knew that the Assyrian empire was at that time the national enemy of his own people. Judgment upon Nineveh would relieve the Assyrian threat to Israel. Conversely, mercy toward Nineveh would increase the danger to Israel. Therefore, Jonah was reluctant to carry any message to Nineveh which might avert God's impending judgment upon that city.

However, at the second call, after undergoing the severe discipline of God, Jonah went to Nineveh. His message was very simple: *"Yet forty days, and Nineveh shall be overthrown"*

(Jonah 3:4). The response of the people of Nineveh was immediate and dramatic. It is described in the next five verses:

> *So the people of Nineveh believed God, and proclaimed a fast, and put on sackcloth, from the greatest of them even to the least of them.*
> *For word came unto the king of Nineveh, and he arose from his throne, and he laid his robe from him, and covered him with sackcloth, and sat in ashes.*
> *And he caused it to be proclaimed and published through Nineveh by the decree of the king and his nobles, saying, Let neither man nor beast, herd nor flock, taste anything: let them not feed, nor drink water:*
> *But let man and beast be covered with sackcloth, and cry mightily unto God: yea, let them turn every one from his evil way, and from the violence that is in their hands.*
> *Who can tell if God will turn and repent, and turn away from his fierce anger, that we perish not?* (Jonah 3:5-9)

There is no other instance in Old Testament history of such profound and universal repentance upon the part of a whole community. All normal activities came to a standstill. The king and the nobles proclaimed a fast, and they themselves set the example. They were followed not merely by all the human inhabitants of Nineveh, but even by the herds and the flocks. The entire city cast itself upon the mercy of God. Words could not paint a more vivid picture. Universal, public fasting became the most complete and appropriate expression of deep inner mourning and self-humbling.

The response of God to Nineveh's fasting is described in the last verse of the chapter: *"And God saw their works, that they turned from their evil way; and God repented of the evil that he had said that he would do unto them; and he did it not."* History records that Nineveh, thus spared at the eleventh hour, continued as a more or less stable and prosperous city for about one hundred fifty years, and was finally destroyed in 612 B.C., as predicted by the later prophets Nahum and Zephaniah.

Principles That Apply Today

God's dealings with Nineveh through Jonah illustrate a principle which is more fully unfolded through the prophet Jeremiah. In the Book of Jeremiah, the Lord says:

> At what instant I shall speak concerning a nation, and concerning a kingdom, to pluck up, and to pull down, and to destroy it;

*If that nation, against whom I have pro-
nounced, turn from their evil, I will repent
of the evil that I thought to do unto them.
And at what instant I shall speak concerning a nation, and concerning a kingdom,
to build and to plant it;
If it do evil in my sight, that it obey not my
voice, then I will repent of the good,
wherewith I said I would benefit them.*
(Jeremiah 18:7-10)

In God's dealings with nations, His promises of blessing and His warnings of judgment
are both alike: they are conditional. Judgment
may be averted—even at the eleventh hour—
by repentance. Conversely, blessing may be
forfeited by disobedience.

By contrasting the destiny of Assyria with
that of the northern kingdom of Israel, we may
discern principles of God's dealings with nations that still apply today.

In the eighth century B.C., the gentile city
of Nineveh received one warning of judgment
from one prophet—Jonah. The whole population responded with universal repentance.
During the same period, the northern kingdom
of Israel heard the repeated warnings of God
not only from Jonah, but from at least four
other prophets—Amos, Hosea, Isaiah, and
Micah. Yet they rejected these prophets and
refused to repent.

What was the outcome? The Assyrian empire, of which Nineveh was the capital, became the instrument of God's judgment upon Israel. In 721 B.C., the kings of Assyria captured and destroyed Samaria, the capital of Israel, and carried away the entire northern kingdom into captivity.

The tragic end of the northern kingdom seems to support the saying, "Familiarity breeds contempt." Israel, with her long history of special revelation from God, heard many prophets and rejected them. Nineveh, without any previous revelation from God, heard one prophet and received him. This lesson from history contains a special warning to those of us who live in lands with long histories of Christian influence and teaching. Let us beware that we do not allow our familiarity with the message to keep us from acknowledging its urgency!

Today, God is speaking once again through His messengers and by His Spirit to cities and to nations. He is calling to repentance, to fasting, to self-humbling. Those who obey will receive the visitation of His mercy, as Nineveh did. Those who reject will receive the visitation of His wrath, as Israel did.

8

Fasting Prepares for God's Latter Rain

All through the Bible, there is a delicate balance between the fulfillment of God's predetermined purposes and the exercise of human free will. On the one hand, the eternal counsels of God, revealed in the prophecies and promises of His Word, are sure of ultimate fulfillment. On the other hand, there are occasions in which God requires the exercise of human faith and human will as an indispensable condition for the fulfillment of His counsels. To understand this balance, and to apply it in prayer, is the essence of true intercession.

135

The Pattern of Daniel's Intercession

An illuminating example of this is found in the intercessory ministry of Daniel. He says:

> *In the first year of his reign* [i.e. the reign of Darius] *I Daniel understood from the books the number of years, whereof the word of the Lord came to Jeremiah that he would accomplish seventy years in the desolations of Jerusalem.*
> *I set my face unto the Lord God, to seek by prayer and supplications, with fasting, and sackcloth, and ashes.* (Daniel 9:2-3)

Daniel was not only a prophet; he was also a student of prophecy. In the course of studying the prophecies of Jeremiah, he discovered the promise to which he here refers: *"For thus saith the Lord, that after seventy years be accomplished at Babylon I will visit you, and perform my good word toward you, in causing you to return to this place* [i.e. the land of Israel]" (Jeremiah 29:10). Daniel knew that the appointed period of seventy years had almost run its course. He therefore understood that the promised hour of deliverance and restoration was near at hand.

In chapter 4 of this book, we referred to the account of Daniel's prayer given in Daniel 6:10. It is evident from the passage that Daniel already made a practice of regular intercession, three times a day, for the restoration of Israel to their own land. Now the revelation from the prophecy of Jeremiah showed him that the time had come for God to answer his prayers. In studying Daniel's response to this revelation, we gain a vital lesson in the ministry of intercession. A carnally-minded person might have interpreted the promise from Jeremiah as a release from further obligations to pray. If God had promised to restore Israel at that time, what further need was there to pray?

Daniel's response was just the opposite. He did not interpret God's promise as a release from his obligation of intercession, but rather as a challenge to seek God with greater intensity and fervency than ever before. This renewed determination is beautifully expressed in his own words: *"I set my face unto the Lord God"* (Daniel 9:3). In the prayer life of each one of us, there comes a time when we have to set our faces. From that moment onward, no discouragement, no distraction, no opposition will be allowed to hold us back, until we have obtained the full assurance of an answer to which God's Word gives us title.

At this point of seeking God with great intensity, Daniel understood that his prayers must be undergirded by fasting. He says, *"I set my face...to seek by prayer and supplications, with fasting, and sackcloth, and ashes."* Sack-cloth and ashes were the accepted outward evidence of mourning. We see once again how closely fasting is associated with mourning.

As we go on to study the actual prayer of Daniel recorded in the succeeding verses, we see how fasting and mourning were in turn associated with self-humbling. By all human standards, Daniel was one of the most right-eous and God-fearing men portrayed in Scrip-ture—yet at no time does he represent himself as more righteous than those for whom he is interceding. He invariably identifies himself with his own people in all their rebellion and backsliding. His cry is, *"We have sinned, and have committed iniquity...O Lord, righteous-ness belongeth unto thee, but unto us confusion of faces"* (vv. 5, 7). Always it is we and us, never they and them. All through to the end of his prayer, Daniel takes his place as one of those justly subject to the righteous judgments of God that had come upon his people.

Thus, Daniel's prayer is made effective by his own **personal involvement**. This is ex-pressed in three ways that are closely related: **by fasting**, by **mourning**, and by **self-humbling**.

In 2 Chronicles, God states the conditions which His people must fulfill for the healing of their land:

If my people, which are called by my name,
shall humble themselves, and pray, and
seek my face, and turn from their wicked
ways; then will I hear from heaven, and
will forgive their sin, and will heal their
land. (2 Chronicles 7:14)

God's requirements are fourfold: that
His people humble themselves, pray, seek
His face, and turn from their wicked
ways. Upon meeting these conditions, God
promises to hear the prayer of His people and
heal their land.

In the example of Daniel now before us,
we learn exactly what is meant by each of
these requirements. Daniel humbled himself;
he prayed; he set himself to seek God's face;
and identifying himself with his people's sins,
he renounced and turned from those sins. In
turn, the outcome proves the faithfulness of
God to fulfill His promise whenever His conditions are met, for it was through Daniel's intercession that restoration came to Israel and
healing to their land.

Of all the great characters in the Bible,
Daniel exemplifies perhaps more clearly than
any other the ministry which is the theme of
this book: shaping history through prayer and
fasting. When Daniel first came to Babylon as
a young man, it was his prayers (combined

with his gift of revelation) that changed the heart of King Nebuchadnezzar, procuring favor and promotion for the Jews in Babylon. Later, near the end of Daniel's life, when the Babylonian empire had been succeeded by that of Medo-Persia, it was the prayer and fasting of Daniel that finally opened the way for the restoration of Israel to their own land. Over a period of nearly seventy years, the main successive changes in the destiny of God's people can be traced to the prayers of Daniel.

From this study of Daniel's intercession, there emerges one lesson of special importance for our theme. The prophecies and the promises of God's Word are never an excuse to cease praying. On the contrary, they are intended to provoke us to pray with increased earnestness and understanding. God reveals to us the purposes which He is working out, not that we may be passive spectators on the sidelines of history, but that we may personally identify ourselves with His purposes, and thus become actively involved in their fulfillment. **Revelation demands involvement**.

Joel's Thrice-Uttered Call

This lesson applies particularly to the latter-day outpouring of the Holy Spirit which is now making an ever-increasing impact in every area of Christendom and in every part of the world. The great prophet of this outpouring is Joel. It is in Joel's prophecy that God reveals His sovereign purpose to send a visitation of His Spirit upon the whole human race:

> *And it shall come to pass afterward, that I will pour out my spirit upon all flesh; and your sons and your daughters shall prophesy, your old men shall dream dreams, your young men shall see visions.*
>
> *(Joel 2:28)*

On the day of Pentecost, when the Holy Spirit was first poured out, this verse of Joel was quoted by Peter:

> *But this is that which was spoken by the prophet Joel;*
> *And it shall come to pass in the last days, saith God, I will pour out of my Spirit upon all flesh: and your sons and your daughters shall prophesy, and your young men shall see visions, and your old men shall dream dreams.* *(Acts 2:16-17)*

Between the passage in Joel and that in Acts, there is one significant difference. Where Joel says, *"It shall come to pass afterward,"* Peter says, *"It shall come to pass in the last days."* Peter applied these words to events that were then taking place. We may thus infer that the day of Pentecost marked the beginning of the period defined in Scripture as *"the last days."* This period of the last days still continues, and will do so until the present age closes. Thus, Peter's words give us a scriptural starting point for the last days.

In this connection, it is important also to note that the outpouring of the Holy Spirit predicted by Joel was to be divided into two main phases: *"the former rain"* and *"the latter rain."* This is stated in Joel 2:23: *"He* [God] *will cause to come down for you the rain, the former rain, and the latter rain in the first month."* The rain is the type, of which the outpoured Holy Spirit is the antitype. In the actual climatic pattern of Israel, the former rain falls at the beginning of winter (about November), and the latter rain falls at the end of winter (about March or April). Thus the latter rain more or less coincides with the Passover, which according to the Jewish religious calendar occurs in the middle of *"the first month"* (see Exodus 12:2).

By transferring this from type to antitype, we arrive at a logical inference: the former rain of the Holy Spirit marks the beginning of the last days, while the latter rain of the Holy Spirit marks the close of the last days. God both begins and ends His dealings with the church on earth by a universal outpouring of

His Holy Spirit. The first rain of the Holy
Spirit fell on the early church. The latter rain
of the Holy Spirit is now falling on the church
worldwide in our days. Such is the implication
of Peter's phrase, *"the last days."*

Now let us turn back to the original version of the prophecy, as given in Joel 2:28:
*"And it shall come to pass afterward, that I will
pour out my spirit upon all flesh."* Where Peter
says *"in the last days,"* Joel says *"afterward."*
In order to understand the total message of
Joel, we must rightly interpret this word *afterward.* What does Joel mean by it? After
what? Obviously he refers to something that
he has said earlier in his prophecy.

If we turn back to the beginning of Joel's
prophecy, we are confronted with a scene of
unrelieved and total desolation. Every part of
the inheritance of God's people is affected. All
is blighted; nothing is fruitful. There is no ray
of hope, no human solution. What does God
tell His people to do? The remedy which God
prescribes is united fasting: *"Sanctify ye a fast,
call a solemn assembly, gather the elders and
all the inhabitants of the land into the house of
the Lord your God, and cry unto the Lord"*
(Joel 1:14).

To sanctify here means *to set apart.* God's
call to fasting must have absolute preeminence. Every other activity, religious or

secular, must take second place. There is particular emphasis upon the elders. The leaders of God's people have a special responsibility in this respect. However, all the inhabitants of the land are included. There must be no exceptions. God's people are required to unite in facing their need. They are called to gather together in fasting, just as they did in the days of Jehoshaphat, of Ezra, and of Esther.

In Joel 2:12, the call is repeated: *"Therefore also now, saith the Lord, turn ye even to me with all your heart, and with fasting, and with weeping, and with mourning."* In hours of crisis such as this, prayer alone will not suffice. Prayer must be accompanied by fasting, weeping, and mourning. (We notice again the very close connections between fasting and mourning.)

In Joel 2:15, the call to fasting comes the third time: *"Blow the trumpet in Zion, sanctify a fast, call a solemn assembly."* Zion is the assembly of God's people. Blowing the trumpet is the most public form of proclamation that is possible. There is nothing private or secret about a fast that is proclaimed in this way. The Bible makes it plain that there are times when fasting is to be publicly proclaimed for all of God's people.

The passage continues:

> *Gather the people, sanctify the congrega-*
> *tion, assemble the elders, gather the chil-*
> *dren, and those that suck the breasts....*
> *Let the priests, the ministers of the Lord,*
> *weep between the porch and the altar.*
> *(Joel 2:16-17)*

Once again, although all the people are involved, there is special emphasis upon the leadership: the priests, the ministers, and the elders. In chapter 6 of this book, we saw that the responsibility of leaders to set the example in fasting is carried over into the New Testament church.

Three times in these verses of Joel, God calls His people to fasting. Then there follows the promise: *"Afterward I will pour out my spirit upon all flesh."* After what? After God's people have obeyed His call to fasting and prayer. Today God's Spirit is being poured out in a measure. There is ample evidence that the time has come for God's *"latter rain."* But as yet, we see only a small fraction of the total outpouring which the Bible clearly predicts. God is waiting for us to meet His require-ments. **It will take united prayer and fast-ing to precipitate the final fullness of the latter rain**.

In this respect our position today is closely parallel to that of Daniel at the beginning of the reign of Darius. He saw God's hand moving in the political situation. He saw from the Scriptures that God's time had come for the restoration of His people. Prompted by this double witness, Daniel gave himself to prayer and fasting. Only in this way could God's promises be brought to their appointed fulfillment.

The central purpose of God in Daniel's day was restoration. God was moving to bring His people back into the inheritance which they had lost through disobedience. The same is true today. The outpouring of the Holy Spirit is God's appointed means of restoration. God declares this in Joel 2:25: *"I will restore to you the years that the locust hath eaten."*

Three-and-a-half centuries ago, the church experienced **reformation**. Today God is no longer concerned with reformation. His purpose is **restoration**. God is moving to restore every area of His people's inheritance to its original condition. The *"former rain"* brought into being a church that satisfied the divine standards of purity, power, and order. The *"latter rain"* will restore the church to the same standards. Then—and only then—will the church be able to fulfill its destiny in the world. This is the end toward which God is now working.

Isaiah's Great Fasting Chapter

It is appropriate to close our study of fasting in the Old Testament by turning to Isaiah chapter 58. This is the great "fasting chapter" of the Old Testament. Isaiah describes two different ways of fasting. In verses 3 through 5, Isaiah describes the kind of fast which is not acceptable to God. Then in verses 6 to12, he describes the kind of fast which is well pleasing to God.

The fault with the first kind of fasting lies mainly in the motives and the attitudes of those practicing it.

> *Behold, in the day of your fast ye find pleasure, and exact all your labors* [or things wherewith ye grieve others].
> *Behold, ye fast for strife and debate, and to smite with the fist of wickedness....*
> *Is it such a fast that I have chosen?...a day for a man...to bow down his head as a bulrush?*　　　　　(Isaiah 58:3-5)

For the people here described, fasting was merely an accepted part of religious ritual. This was the kind of fasting practiced by the Pharisees in Jesus' day. There was no real repentance or self-humbling. On the contrary, they continued with all their normal secular

affairs and retained all their evil attitudes of
greed, selfishness, pride, and oppression. The
"bow[ing] *down of the head as a bulrush"* is a
very vivid description of certain forms of
prayer still practiced by some orthodox Jews,
in which they rock to and fro with their torsos,
mechanically repeating set prayers of which
they scarcely understand the meaning.

On the other hand, the kind of fast which
is well pleasing to God springs from motives
and attitudes that are totally different. In
verse six, Isaiah defines the motives behind
this kind of fasting: *"To loose the bands of
wickedness, to undo the heavy burdens, and to
let the oppressed go free, and that ye break every
yoke."* Scripture and experience alike confirm
that there are many bands that cannot be
loosed, many burdens that cannot be undone,
many yokes that cannot be broken, and many
oppressed who will never go free until God's
people—and especially their leaders—obey
God's call to fasting and prayer.

Isaiah continues by describing the
attitudes toward other people—and especially
toward the needy and the oppressed—which
are part of the kind of fasting approved by
God. *"Is it not to deal thy bread to the hungry,
and that thou bring the poor that are cast out to
thy house? when thou seest the naked, that thou
cover him; and that thou hide not thyself from*

thine own flesh?" (v. 7). Fasting of this kind must be united with sincere and practical charity in our dealings with those around us— particularly those who need our help in material and financial matters.

Isaiah once again warns against the wrong attitudes associated with the kind of fasting that is not acceptable to God, and contrasts these attitudes with true, practical charity.

> *If thou take away from the midst of thee the yoke, the putting forth of the finger, and speaking vanity;*
> *And if thou draw out thy soul to the hungry, and satisfy the afflicted soul.*
> *(Isaiah 58:9-10)*

"The yoke, the putting forth of the finger, and speaking vanity" may be summed up in three words: **legalism, criticism, and insincerity**.

Now let us consider the blessings promised by Isaiah to those who practice the kind of fasting acceptable to God. These blessings are listed in successive stages. First, Isaiah describes those of health and righteousness:

> *Then shall thy light break forth as the morning, and thine health spring forth speedily: and thy righteousness shall go before thee; the glory of the Lord shall be thy reward.* *(Isaiah 58:8)*

This is in harmony with the promise of Malachi 4:2: *"But unto you that fear my name shall the Sun of righteousness arise with healing in his wings."* The context in Malachi indicates a special application to the period just prior to the close of the present age.

In verse nine, Isaiah describes the blessing of answered prayer: *"Then thou shalt call, and the Lord shall answer; thou shalt cry, and he shall say, Here I am."* Here is God at man's disposal, ready to answer every petition and to supply every need.

Next, Isaiah describes the blessings of guidance and fruitfulness:

> *Then shall thy light rise in obscurity, and thy darkness be as the noon day:*
> *And the Lord shall guide thee continually, and satisfy thy soul in drought, and make fat thy bones: and thou shalt be like a watered garden and like a spring of waters, whose waters fail not.   (Isaiah 58:10-11)*

Finally, Isaiah describes the blessings of restoration:

> *And they that be of thee shall build the old waste places: thou shalt raise up the foundations of many generations; thou shalt be called, The repairer of the breach, The restorer of paths to dwell in.   (Isaiah 58:12)*

Like Joel, Isaiah points to a close connection between fasting and the restoration of God's people. Isaiah closes his message on fasting with this theme: *"building the old waste places...repairing the breach...restoring paths to dwell in."* This work of restoration is the purpose of God for His people at this time. The divinely appointed means to accomplish it is prayer and fasting.

In the light of this clear and consistent message from the Word of God, each one of us is brought to a place of personal decision. In Ezekiel 22:30, God says: *"I sought for a man among them, that should make up the hedge, and stand in the gap before me for the land, that I should not destroy it."* Again today God is looking for a man like that. Will you offer yourself to God for this purpose? Will you give yourself to prayer and fasting? Will you join yourself in fellowship with others of like vision and determination, and with them unite in special periods of prayer and fasting?

Let us sanctify a fast! Let us call a solemn assembly! Let us gather together!

9

Practical Guidelines for Fasting

For many Christians today—if not for most—the prospect of fasting is unfamiliar and somewhat frightening. Often, after I have preached in a public meeting on fasting, people have come up to me with questions such as: "How do I start fasting?" "Are there any special dangers to guard against?" "Can't you give me some practical hints?"

Fasting Is Similar to Prayer

Nearly all those who ask such questions are already familiar in some measure with the practice of prayer. Therefore it is helpful to begin by pointing out some of the ways in which fasting is similar to prayer.

Every responsible Christian has to cultivate his personal prayer life on a regular basis. Most Christians find it practical to set aside a definite time each day for personal prayer. Quite frequently, this is a period in the early morning before the normal secular activities of the day begin. Others find it better to devote the close of the day to prayer. Some combine both morning and evening. For each believer, this is settled by personal convenience and by the individual leading of the Holy Spirit.

However, in addition to these regular periods of prayer, almost every Christian finds that there are times when the Holy Spirit calls to special seasons of prayer. These may be provoked by some urgent crisis or by some serious problem that has not been resolved by regular daily prayer. These special seasons of prayer are often more intense or more prolonged than the regular prayer period each day.

The same principles apply to fasting. Every Christian who decides to make fasting a part of his personal spiritual discipline would be wise to set aside one or more specific periods each week for this purpose. In this way, fasting becomes a part of regular spiritual discipline in just the same way as prayer. However, in addition to these regular weekly periods of fasting, it is likely that there will also be special occasions when the Holy Spirit calls to fasting that is more intensive and more prolonged.

It is remarkable how quickly the body will adjust itself to a pattern of regular fasting. From 1949 through 1956, I pastored a congregation in London, England. During these years my wife and I normally observed Thursday as a day of fasting each week. We discovered that our stomachs became "set" to this day, in much the same way that an alarm clock is set to go off at a certain hour. When Thursday came, even if we happened to forget what day of the week it was, our stomachs would not make their normal demands for food. I remember Lydia saying to me on one occasion, "It must be Thursday, I have no appetite this morning!"

In the early days of the Methodist movement, there was strong emphasis upon regular fasting. John Wesley himself made this a part of his own personal discipline. He taught that the early church practiced fasting on Wednesday and Friday of each week, and he exhorted all Methodists of his day to do the same. In fact, he would not ordain to the Methodist ministry any man who would not undertake to fast until 4 P.M. each Wednesday and Friday.

Of course, in the case of both prayer and fasting, we need to guard against any form of legalistic bondage. In Galatians 5:18, Paul says, *"But if ye be led of the Spirit, ye are not under the law."* For the Christian who is led by the Holy Spirit, neither prayer nor fasting should ever become a fixed, legal requirement such as was imposed on Israel under the law of Moses. A Christian may therefore feel perfectly free at any time to change his patterns of prayer and of fasting, as circumstances may require or as the Holy Spirit may direct. He should never allow this to bring him under any sense of guilt or self-condemnation.

In chapter 6 of this book, we saw that, in the Sermon on the Mount, Jesus used the same language about fasting that He used about prayer. He gave instructions for individual prayer: *"When thou* [singular] *prayest...."* He also gave instructions for collective prayer: *"When ye* [plural] *pray...."* Likewise, He gave instructions for both individual and collective fasting. *"When thou* [singular] *fastest..."* indicates the individual. *"When ye* [plural] *fast..."* applies to the group meeting together.

Christians are familiar with the practice of coming together in a group for public prayer. In most churches, the "prayer meeting" is a part of the normal weekly routine. There is just as much scriptural precedent for coming together in a group for public fasting. In chapters 7 and 8 of this book, we examined a whole series of instances in the Old Testament where God called His people together for collective, public fasting. In chapter 6, we saw from the New Testament that in the early church also collective fasting was practiced by whole congregations, with the leaders setting the example.

People sometimes object that Jesus warned His disciples against fasting in public. They quote Matthew:

> *But thou, when thou fastest, anoint thine head, and wash thy face;*
> *That thou appear not unto men to fast, but unto thy Father which seeth in secret: and thy Father, which seeth in secret, shall reward thee openly.   (Matthew 6:17-18)*

We have already pointed out that Jesus is speaking here in the singular, to the individual. This is logical. An individual believer, who fasts by himself, has no need to make his fasting public.

However, in the preceding verse, Jesus speaks in the plural about collective fasting:

> *Moreover when ye fast, be not, as the hypocrites, of a sad countenance: for they disfigure their faces, that they may appear*

> *unto men to fast. Verily I say unto you,*
> *They have their reward.   (Matthew 6:16)*

In this verse, Jesus warns against unnecessary ostentation, but He does not require that fasting be done in secret. This is logical also. Obviously, people cannot come together for collective fasting unless it is arranged by some form of public announcement. This necessarily rules out secrecy.

Without a doubt, the devil is behind this theory that Christians must only fast in secret. It deprives God's people of the most powerful weapon in their whole armory—that of united, public fasting. Those who speak against public fasting usually emphasize the need for "humility." But in this context so-called humility is really a polite religious name for unbelief or disobedience.

Having established these basic principles which apply both to prayer and to fasting, we may now turn more specifically to fasting. Over the years, on the basis of personal experience, I have arrived at a number of practical guidelines that are designed to produce the maximum benefit from fasting. These are set forth briefly here. For convenience, we will deal first with individual fasting and then with collective fasting.

Guidelines for Individual Fasting

1. Enter into fasting with positive faith. God requires faith of this kind in all who seek Him. *"But without faith it is impossible to please him: for he that cometh to God must believe that he is, and that he is a rewarder of them that diligently seek him"* (Hebrews 11:6). If you determine to seek God diligently by fasting, you have a scriptural right to expect that God will reward you. In Matthew 6:18, Jesus gives this promise to the believer who fasts with the right motives: *"Thy Father, which seeth in secret, shall reward thee openly."*

2. Remember: *"Faith cometh by hearing, and hearing by the word of God"* (Romans 10:17). Your fasting should be based upon the conviction that God's Word enjoins this as a part of normal Christian discipline. Hopefully, the preceding three chapters will have helped you to arrive at this conviction.

3. Do not wait for some emergency to drive you to fasting. It is better to begin fasting when you are spiritually "up," rather than when you are "down." The law of progress in God's kingdom is: *"from strength to strength"*

(Psalm 84:7); *"from faith to faith"* (Romans 1:17); *"from glory to glory"* (2 Corinthians 3:18).

4. In the beginning, do not set yourself too long a period of fasting. If you are fasting for the first time, omit one or two meals. Then move on gradually to longer periods, such as a day or two days. It is better to begin by setting a short period as your objective and achieving it. If you set too long a time at the outset and fail to meet it, you may become discouraged and give up.

5. During your fast, give plenty of time to Bible study. Where possible, read a portion of Scripture before each period of prayer. The Psalms are particularly helpful. Read them aloud, identifying yourself with the prayers, the praises and the confessions contained in them.

6. It is often helpful to set certain specific objectives in your fasting and to make a written list of these. If you keep the lists that you make and turn back to them after an interval of time, your faith will be strengthened when you see how many of your objectives have been achieved.

7. Avoid religious ostentation and boastfulness. Apart from special periods of

prayer or other spiritual activity, your life and conduct while fasting should be as normal and unpretentious as possible. This is the essence of the warnings given by Jesus in Matthew 6:16-18. Remember that boasting is excluded by the law of faith. (See Romans 3:27.) Fasting does not earn you any merit badges from God. It is part of your duty as a committed Christian. Bear in mind the warning of Jesus in Luke 17:10: *"So likewise ye, when ye shall have done all those things which are commanded you, say, We are unprofitable servants: we have done that which was our duty to do."*

8. Each time you fast, keep a watchful check on your motives. Take time to read Isaiah 58:1-12 once again. Note the motives and attitudes which are unpleasing to God. Then study the motives and objectives which are pleasing to God. Your own motives and objectives should line up with these.

Physical Aspects of Fasting

When practiced with due care and sense, fasting is beneficial to the physical body. Here are some points to observe, if you wish to obtain the physical benefits of fasting.

1. Remember that *"your body is the temple of the Holy Spirit"* (1 Corinthians 6:19). It pleases God when you take proper care of your body, seeking to make it a clean and healthy temple for His Spirit. Health is one of the specific benefits promised to fasting when it is properly practiced (Isaiah 58:8).

2. If you are on regular medication, or if you suffer from some kind of wasting disease, such as diabetes or tuberculosis, it is wise to obtain medical advice before entering into any fast that extends beyond a meal or two.

3. In the early period of a fast, you may experience unpleasant physical symptoms, such as dizziness, headache, or nausea. Usually these are indications that your fasting is overdue and that you need the purifying physical action of fasting in various areas of your body. Do not allow physical discomfort to deter you. *"Set your face"* (Ezekiel 4:3 RSV), and go through with the fast that you planned. After the first day or two, these unpleasant physical reactions usually subside.

4. Remember that hunger is partly a matter of habit. In the early stages of a fast, hunger will probably return at each normal mealtime. But if you hold out, the sensation of hunger will pass away without your having eaten anything. Sometimes you can fool your stomach by drinking a glass of water instead of eating.

5. Guard against constipation. Before and after fasting, choose meals that will help you in this respect, such as: fresh fruit or fruit juices; dried figs, prunes or apricots; oatmeal, etc.

6. During a fast some people drink only water. Others take various kinds of fluid, such as fruit juices, broth, or skim milk. It is wise to abstain from strong stimulants such as tea or coffee. Do not come under bondage to other people's theories. Work out for yourself the particular pattern of fasting which suits you best as an individual.

7. It is scriptural to abstain at times from fluids as well as from solid food. But do not abstain from fluids for a period exceeding seventy-two hours. This was the limit set by Esther and her maidens (Esther 4:16). To go over seventy-two hours without fluids can

have disastrous physical effects. It is true that Moses twice spent forty days without eating or drinking. (See Deuteronomy 9:9-18.) However, Moses was then on a supernatural plane in the immediate presence of God. Unless you are on the same supernatural plane, do not attempt to follow Moses' example.

8. Break your fast gradually. Begin with meals that are light and easy to digest. The longer you have fasted, the more careful you need to be about breaking your fast. At this point you will need to exercise watchful self-control. Eating too heavily after a fast can produce serious physical discomfort and can nullify the physical benefits of fasting.

9. During any fast that exceeds two days, your stomach will shrink. Do not over-expand it again. If you have been prone to eat too heavily, guard against going back to this habit. If you train yourself to eat more lightly, your stomach will adjust itself accordingly.

Guidelines for Collective Fasting

For periods of collective fasting, all the guidelines given above for individual fasting will normally continue to apply. In addition, here are a few special points to observe in connection with collective fasting.

1. In Matthew 18:19, Jesus emphasizes the special power that is released when believers *"agree"* together in prayer. To this end, all those participating in a collective fast should do everything in their power to achieve and to maintain agreement with each other.

2. People participating in a collective fast should make a commitment to pray specifically for each other during the period of the fast.

3. A meeting place should be chosen where those participating in the fast can come together at times mutually agreed upon.

A Record of God's Faithfulness

It is appropriate to bring this chapter to a close with a personal testimony to God's faithfulness. Over the past fifty years or more, I have from time to time devoted myself to periods of special prayer and fasting. For some of these I set specific objectives in prayer and kept records, which are still available.

As I look back now over these records, I am frequently amazed to see how many times and in how many ways God has answered my prayers. Sometimes there is a long interval between the date on which I recorded a specific prayer request and the date on which it was answered. Quite frequently, I recorded prayer requests and later forgot about them. But looking back through my records, I find that God did not forget. In His way and in His season, God answered even these requests which I myself had forgotten.

As I write, I have before me the record of a special period of prayer and fasting which I undertook in 1951. According to my record, this period began on July 24 and extended through August 16—a total of twenty-four days. At that time, I was engaged in full-time pastoral ministry. I continued to discharge all my normal duties, which included ministering at five services each week and also three street meetings.

I am amused to observe that, for this particular period, I wrote out the complete list of my special prayer objectives in New Testament Greek. The things for which I was praying were so intimate and so sacred to me that I wanted to keep the list known only to God and to myself. For this reason I made it in a language not understood by most people today!

I divided up this particular list into five main sections:

A. My own spiritual needs
B. Needs of my family
C. Needs of the church
D. Needs of my country (Great Britain)
E. Needs of the world

Many of the things I prayed for are still too personal for me to divulge. However, there are points about which I feel free to write.

As I look through the various requests made on behalf of my family, I can see that every one of them has definitely been answered. The last request in this section was for the salvation of my mother. This took place about fourteen years later.

Among the requests which I made for myself was one for the exercise of four specific spiritual gifts. At that time, I scarcely understood the nature of the gifts which I was seeking. Yet today I can say that all these four gifts are regularly manifested in my ministry.

The requests I made for the church and the world are in a large measure being answered by the worldwide outpouring of the Holy Spirit that is now taking place. However, if God's people will seek Him more earnestly in prayer and fasting on a wider scale, I believe that we shall see a move of the Holy Spirit throughout the entire world, such as history has yet to record. Indeed, we shall see fulfilled the prophecy of Habakkuk 2:14: *"For the earth shall be filled with the knowledge of the glory of the Lord, as the waters cover the sea."*

Of my requests for Britain, only a small fraction have so far been answered. However, in 1953—two years after this particular period of fasting—God awakened me one night and spoke to me audibly. The first promise that He gave me was, "There shall be a great revival in the United States and Great Britain." This revival is already underway in the United States, and there are evidences that it is beginning also in Britain. I have no doubt in my heart that God's promise for Britain will be fulfilled. By His grace, I expect to witness it.

As I meditate on these personal experiences of God's power and faithfulness, I find myself spontaneously echoing Paul's words:

> *Now unto him that is able to do exceeding abundantly, above all that we ask or think, according to the power that worketh in us; Unto him be glory in the church by Christ Jesus throughout all ages, world without end. Amen.* (Ephesians 3:20-21)

10

Laying a Foundation by Fasting

In 1970 and 1971, the city of Plymouth, Massachusetts, celebrated the three hundred fiftieth anniversary of the landing of the pilgrims at that point on the coast of America. A special committee was appointed by the city to organize various kinds of celebration that were appropriate to the occasion. This committee paid me the honor of inviting me to give a series of addresses in the Church of the Pilgrimage in the city of Plymouth. During my visit there, two members of the committee were kind enough to show me the main places of historical interest and also to introduce me to some of the original records of the period of the pilgrims. In this way, I became acquainted for the first time with the history, *Of Plymouth Plantation,* written by William Bradford.

Background of the Pilgrims

Having been educated in Britain, I do not recall ever having learned anything at school about the pilgrims. The phrase, "Pilgrim Fathers," commonly used by Americans, had created in my mind a vague impression of severe old men with long white beards, probably attired in dark formal clothing similar to that associated with ministers of religion. I was surprised to discover that the majority of the pilgrims at the time of their arrival in America were still young men and women. For example, William Bradford was thirty-one years old in 1621, when he was first appointed governor of the colony. Most of the other pilgrims were of about the same age or younger. As portrayed in wax in the historical tableau on board the replica of the Mayflower in Plymouth harbor, Bradford and his companions reminded me not a little of the Jesus People who emerged on this continent in the 1960s.

As I studied Bradford's own firsthand account of the founding of Plymouth Colony and of its early struggles, I developed a strong sense of spiritual kinship with him and his fellow pilgrims. I discovered that their whole way of life was based upon the systematic study and application of the Scriptures. With the main conclusions and convictions to which this study led them, I found myself in complete accord. In fact, they are in close agreement with some of the main themes developed in this book.

Having obtained my own degrees in the University of Cambridge and having held a fellowship at King's College, Cambridge, I was particularly interested to see how many of the pilgrims' spiritual leaders had received their education at Cambridge. Three of those most closely associated with the pilgrims' story were Richard Clyfton, John Robinson, and William Brewster. Clyfton was the elder of the original congregation at Scrooby, in England. Robinson was the elder of the pilgrims' congregation at Leyden, in Holland. Brewster was the elder who actually traveled over on the *Mayflower* and became the chief spiritual leader of the original colony in Plymouth. All three of these men received their education at Cambridge.

During the months that followed my visit to Plymouth, I traveled widely and conducted meetings in various parts of the United States. I began to share with those I met some of my stimulating discoveries from Bradford's book, *Of Plymouth Plantation*. To my surprise, I encountered almost complete and universal ignorance of the whole subject. Many people of at least average education, born and raised in the United States, confessed that they had never heard of the book. A few acknowledged that they had heard of the book, but none, as I recall, had actually read it.

For this reason, I feel that I need offer no apology for quoting from Bradford's book various passages that relate to the theme of our present study. All the quotations that follow are taken from the edition published by Modern Library Books, with an introduction and notes by Samuel E. Morison.

The whole course of Bradford's life was determined by spiritual experiences of his boyhood and early manhood. In Morison's introduction to his edition of Bradford's book, these early experiences are briefly described as follows:

> William Bradford was born at Austerfield, Yorkshire, in the early spring of 1590....
> At the age of twelve he became a constant reader of the Bible—the Geneva version that he generally quotes—and when still a lad he was so moved by the Word as to join a group of Puritans who met for prayer and discussion at the house of William Brewster in the nearby village of Scrooby. When this group, inspired by the Rev. Richard Clyfton, organized itself as a

separate Congregational Church in 1606, Bradford joined it despite "the wrath of his uncles" and the "scoff of his neighbors." From that date until his death half a century later, Bradford's life revolved around that of his church or congregation, first in Scrooby, next in the Low Countries and finally in New England.

Restoration, Not Reformation

Although the pilgrims were initially associated with the Puritans, there were important differences between them. Both saw the need of religious reform, but they differed concerning the means by which reform was to be achieved. The Puritans determined to remain within the established church and to impose reform from within—by compulsion, if necessary. The pilgrims sought liberty for themselves, but declined to use the machinery of secular government to enforce their views upon others. These differing points of view are expressed in the following passage from Leonard Bacon's *Genesis of the New England Churches*:

In the Old World on the other side of the ocean, the Puritan was a Nationalist, believing that a Christian nation is a Christian church, and demanding that the

Church of England should be thoroughly
reformed; while the Pilgrim was a Separa-
tist, not only from the Anglican Prayer
Book and Queen Elizabeth's episcopacy,
but from all national churches....

The Pilgrim wanted liberty for himself and his wife and little ones, and for his
brethren, to walk with God in a Christian
life as the rules and motives of such a life
were revealed to him from God's Word.
For that he went into exile; for that he
crossed the ocean; for that he made his
home in a wilderness. The Puritan's idea
was not liberty, but right government in
church and state—such government as
should not only permit him, but also com-
pel other men to walk in the right way.

The difference between Puritans and pilgrims could be expressed in the two words *reformation* and *restoration*. **The Puritans
sought to reform the church as it existed
in their day. The pilgrims believed that
the ultimate purpose of God was to restore the church to its original condition,
as portrayed in the New Testament**. This
shines forth very clearly in the first paragraph
of the first chapter of Bradford's book, where
he expresses the pilgrims' vision of restoration
in the following words:

...the churches of God revert to their ancient purity and recover their primitive
[i.e. original] order, liberty and beauty.

(p. 3)

Later in this chapter, Bradford returns to
this theme when he declares the pilgrims' purpose:

[They labored] to have the right worship
of God and discipline of Christ established
in the church, according to the simplicity
of the gospel, without the mixture of
men's inventions; and to have and be
ruled by the laws of God's Word, dis-
pensed in those offices, and by those officers of Pastors, Teachers and Elders, etc.,
according to the Scriptures. (p. 6)

With this purpose in view, the original
group of believers in Nottinghamshire, Lin-
colnshire, and Yorkshire:

...joined themselves (by a covenant of the
Lord) into a church estate, in the fellowship of the gospel, to walk in all His ways
made known, or to be made known unto
them, according to their best endeavors,
whatsoever it should cost them, the Lord
assisting them. (p. 9)

Later when the congregation moved to Leyden, in Holland, Bradford described their way of life there:

> ...they came as near the primitive [original] pattern of the first churches as any other church[es] of these later times have done.　　　　　　　　　(p. 19)

Again in his fourth chapter, Bradford describes the main motive of the pilgrims in undertaking their journey to America:

> Lastly (and which was not least), a great hope and inward zeal they had of laying some good foundation...for the propagating and advancing of the gospel of the kingdom of Christ in those remote parts of the world; yea, though they should be but even as steppingstones unto others for the performing of so great a work.　　(p. 25)

Public Days of Fasting Proclaimed

One distinctive practice employed by the pilgrims to achieve their spiritual goals was that of united public prayer and fasting. There are various references to this in Bradford's book. One of the most poignant passages describes the pilgrims' preparation for their departure from Leyden:

So being ready to depart, they had a day of solemn humiliation, their pastor [John Robinson] taking his text from Ezra 8:21: *"And there at the river, by Ahava, I proclaimed a fast, that we might humble ourselves before our God, and seek of him a right way for us, and for our children, and for all our substance."* Upon which he [Robinson] spent a good part of the day very profitably and suitable to their present occasion; the rest of the time was spent in pouring out prayers to the Lord with great fervency, mixed with abundance of tears.   (p. 47)

Bradford's use of the word *humiliation* indicates that the pilgrims understood the scriptural connection (explained in chapters 6 through 8 of this book) between fasting and self-humbling. Robinson's choice of the text from Ezra is singularly appropriate. Both in motivation and in experience, there is a close parallel between the pilgrims' embarking on their journey to the New World and Ezra's company of exiles returning from Babylon to Jerusalem to help in the restoration of the temple.

The end of Robinson's address is given by Edward Winslow in Verna M. Hall's *Christian History of the Constitution*:

We are now ere long to part asunder, and the Lord knoweth whether he [Robinson] should live to see our face again. But whether the Lord had appointed it or not, he charged us before God and His blessed angels, to follow him no further than he followed Christ; and if God should reveal anything to us by any other instrument of His, to be as ready to receive it, as ever we were to receive any truth by his ministry; for he was very confident the Lord had more truth and light yet to break forth out of His holy Word. He took occasion also miserably to bewail the state and condition of the Reformed churches who were come to a period [standstill] in religion, and would go no further than the instruments of their reformation [i.e. those who had been leaders in the Reformation].

As for example, the Lutherans, they could not be drawn to go beyond what Luther saw; for whatever part of God's will He had further imparted and revealed to Calvin, they [the Lutherans] will rather die than embrace it. And so also, saith he, you see the Calvinists, they stick where he [Calvin] left them, a misery much to be lamented; for though they were precious shining lights in their times, yet God had not revealed His whole will to them; and were they now living, saith he, they would be as ready and willing to embrace further light, as that they had received.

Here also he put us in mind of our church covenant, at least that part of it whereby we promise and covenant with God and one another to receive whatsoever light or truth shall be made known to us from His written Word; but withal [he] exhorted us to take heed what we received for truth, and well to examine and compare it and weigh it with other Scriptures of truth before we received it. For saith he, it is not possible [that] the Christian world should come so lately [recently] out of such thick antichristian darkness, and that full perfection of knowledge should break forth at once. (p. 184)

John Robinson's message on this occasion sums up the essence of the pilgrims' theological position. This is indicated by their very choice of the name *pilgrims*. They did not claim to have arrived at a final understanding of all truth. They were on a pilgrimage, looking for the further revelation of truth that lay ahead as they walked in obedience to truth already received.

Bradford himself believed firmly that he and his companions were in the same line of spiritual pilgrimage as the saints of the Old and New Testaments, and he habitually resorted to the language of the Bible to express his feelings and reactions. In chapter 9, he describes the arrival of the *Mayflower* at Cape Cod, and the many dangers and hardships which the pilgrims encountered. He concludes the chapter with this:

> What could now sustain them but the Spirit of God and His grace? May not the children of these fathers rightly say: "Our fathers were Englishmen which came over this great ocean, and were ready to perish in this wilderness; but they cried unto the Lord, and He heard their voice and looked on their adversity." [This is Bradford's own paraphrase of Deuteronomy 26:5, 7.]
>
> "Let them therefore praise the Lord, because He is good: and His mercies endure forever. Yea, let them which have been redeemed of the Lord, shew how He hath delivered them from the hand of the oppressor. When they wandered in the desert wilderness out of the way, and found no city to dwell in, both hungry and thirsty, their soul was overwhelmed in them. Let them confess before the Lord His lovingkindness and His wonderful works before the sons of men." [This is Bradford's version of Psalm 107:1-5, 8.]

It is not possible to quote the many instances of answered prayer that Bradford records, but there is one further instance of a public fast that must be mentioned. In the summer of 1623, the corn crop which the pilgrims had so carefully planted was threatened:

> ...by a great drought which continued from the third week in May, till about the middle of July, without any rain and with great heat for the most part, insomuch as the corn began to wither away....it began to languish sore, and some of the drier grounds were parched like withered hay....Upon which they set apart a solemn day of humiliation to seek the Lord by humble and fervent prayer....And He was pleased to give them a gracious and speedy answer, both to their own and the Indians' admiration [i.e. amazement]....For all the morning, and greatest part of the day, it was clear weather and very hot, and not a cloud or any sign of rain to be seen; yet toward evening it began to overcast, and shortly after to rain with such sweet and gentle showers as gave them cause of rejoicing and blessing God....

Normally, if rain had fallen at all in such conditions, it would have been in the form of a thunderstorm, which would have beaten down the corn and destroyed the last hope of a harvest. But on this occasion, Bradford goes on to relate:

It came without either wind or thunder or
any violence, and by degrees in that abundance as that the earth was thoroughly...
soaked therewith. Which did so apparently
revive and quicken the decayed corn and
other fruits, as was wonderful to see, and
made the Indians astonished to behold.
And afterwards the Lord sent them such
seasonable showers, with interchange of
fair warm weather as, through His blessing, caused a fruitful and liberal harvest....
For which mercy, in time convenient, they
also set apart a day of thanksgiving.

(pp. 131-2)

This practice of setting aside special days
of prayer and fasting became an accepted part
of the life of Plymouth Colony. On November
15, 1636, a law was passed allowing the governor and his assistants "to command solemn
days of humiliation by fasting, etc. and also for
thanksgiving as occasion shall be offered."

In chapter 8 of this book, we examined the
promises given in Isaiah to those who practice
the kind of fasting approved by God, and we
saw that these come to their climax in this
verse:

*And they that be of thee shall build the old
waste places: thou shalt raise up the foundations of many generations; and thou*

> *shalt be called, The repairer of the breach,*
> *The restorer of paths to dwell in.*
> *(Isaiah 58:12)*

History has demonstrated that the results of fasting promised in this verse were achieved by the pilgrims. Both spiritually and politically, they *"raise*[d] *up the foundations of many generations."* Three-and-a-half centuries later, the people of the United States are still building on the foundations which the pilgrims laid.

11

Fasts Proclaimed in American History

The pattern set by the pilgrims of proclaiming public days of fasting was followed in subsequent generations both by the governing bodies and by the most famous individual leaders of the American people. The following are some documented examples of this practice.

George Washington and the Assembly of Virginia

In May of 1774, news was received in Williamsburg, Virginia, that the British Parliament had ordered an embargo on the Port of Boston, Massachusetts, to become effective on June 1. Immediately, the Burgesses of Virginia passed a resolution protesting this act and setting aside the day appointed for the commencement of the embargo—June 1—as a day of fasting, humiliation, and prayer.

The following is the main part of the resolution, as recorded in the *Journals Of The House Of Burgesses Of Virginia, 1773-1776*, edited by John Pendleton Kennedy:

Tuesday, the 24th of May, 14 Geo. III. 1774

This House, being deeply impressed with Apprehension of the great Dangers, to be derived to British America, from the hostile Invasion of the City of Boston, in our Sister Colony of Massachusetts Bay, whose Commerce and Harbour are, on the first Day of June next, to be stopped by an armed Force, deem it highly necessary that the said first Day of June be set apart, by the Members of this House, as a Day of Fasting, Humiliation, and Prayer, devoutly to implore the Divine Interposition, for averting the heavy Calamity which threatens Destruction to our civil Rights, and the Evils of civil War; to give us one Heart and one Mind to oppose, by all just and proper Means, every Injury to American Rights....

Ordered, therefore, that the Members of this House do attend in their Places, at the Hour of ten in the Forenoon, on the

*said first Day of June next, in order to
proceed with the Speaker, and the Mace, to
the Church in this City, for the Purposes
aforesaid; and that the Reverend Mr. Price
be appointed to read Prayers, and the
Reverend Mr. Gwatkin, to preach a
Sermon, suitable to the Occasion.*

That this resolution was adhered to is attested by no less a person than George Washington, who wrote in his diary for that first day of June: "Went to Church and fasted all Day." (*The Diaries of George Washington, 1748-1799*, edited by John C. Fitzpatrick.)

The church referred to in the resolution and in Washington's diary was the Parish Church of Bruton in the city of Williamsburg.

Washington not only believed in praying for divine intervention, but he also believed in acknowledging such intervention when prayer was answered. On January 1, 1795, as president of the United States, Washington issued a proclamation setting aside February 19, 1795 for national thanksgiving and prayer. The following is part of the proclamation's text:

When we review the calamities which afflict so many other nations, the present condition of the United States affords much matter of consolation and satisfaction....In such a state of things it is, in an especial manner, our duty as a people, with devout reverence and affectionate gratitude, to acknowledge our many and great obligations to Almighty God, and to implore Him to continue and confirm the blessings we experience.

Deeply penetrated with this sentiment, I, GEORGE WASHINGTON, President of the United States, do recommend to all religious societies and denominations, and to all persons whomsoever within the United States, to set apart and observe Thursday, the nineteenth day of February next, as a day of public Thanksgiving and Prayer; and on that day to meet together, and render their sincere and hearty thanks to the great Ruler of Nations for the manifest and signal mercies which distinguish our lot as a Nation...and at the same time, humbly and fervently to beseech the kind author of these blessings graciously to prolong them to us,—to imprint on our hearts a deep and solemn sense of our obligations to Him for them—to teach us rightly to estimate their immense value—to preserve us from the arrogance of prosperity, and from hazarding the advantages we enjoy by delusive pursuits—to dispose us to merit the continuance of his favors, by not abusing them, by our gratitude for them, and by a correspondent conduct as citizens and as men; to render this country more and more a safe and propitious asylum for the unfortunate of other countries; to extend among us true and useful knowledge; to diffuse and establish habits of sobriety, order, morality, and piety, and finally to impart all the blessings we possess, or ask for ourselves, to the whole family of mankind.

(Appendix no. 5, Volume 11, U.S. Statutes At Large.)

Fasts Proclaimed by Adams and Madison

Under the next president, John Adams, the United States came to the verge of open war with France. On March 23, 1798, Adams proclaimed May 9, 1798 as a day of solemn humiliation, fasting and prayer. The following is part of his proclamation:

As the safety and prosperity of nations ultimately and essentially depend on the protection and the blessing of Almighty God, and the national acknowledgment of this truth is not only an indispensable duty which the people owe to Him, but a duty whose natural influence is favorable to the promotion of that morality and piety, without which social happiness cannot exist, nor the blessings of free government be enjoyed...and as the United States of America are, at present, placed in a hazardous and afflictive situation, by the unfriendly disposition, conduct, and demands of a Foreign Power (i.e. France)....Under these considerations it has appeared to me that the duty of imploring the mercy and benediction of Heaven on our country, demands, at this time, a special attention from its inhabitants.

I have, therefore, thought fit to recommend and I do hereby recommend that Wednesday, the ninth day of May next, be observed throughout the United States, as a day of Solemn Humiliation, Fasting, and Prayer: That the Citizens of these States, abstaining on that day from their customary worldly occupations, offer their devout addresses to the Father of Mercies, agreeably to those forms or methods which they have severally adopted as the most suitable and becoming: That all Religious Congregations do, with the deepest humility, acknowledge before God the manifold sins and transgressions with which we are justly chargeable as individuals and as a nation, beseeching Him at the same time of His infinite grace through the Redeemer of the World, freely to remit all our offenses, and to incline us, by His Holy Spirit, to that sincere Repentance and Reformation, which may afford us reason to hope for His inestimable favor and Heavenly Benediction: That it be made the subject of particular and earnest supplication, that our

*country may be protected from all the dangers
which threaten it: That our civil and religious
privileges may be preserved inviolate, and
perpetuated to the latest generations....*

(Appendix no. 7, Volume 11, U.S. Statutes At Large.)

Under the fourth president, James Madison, the United States found itself at war with Britain. In face of this situation, the two Houses of Congress passed a joint resolution desiring a day of public humiliation, fasting, and prayer. In response, Madison set apart January 12, 1815 for this purpose. His proclamation opened as follows:

*The two houses of the National Legislature
having, by a joint resolution expressed their
desire that, in the present time of public calamity and war, a day may be recommended to be
observed by the people of the United States as a
day of public humiliation and fasting, and of
prayer to Almighty God for the safety and welfare of these States, his blessing on their arms
and a speedy restoration of peace: I have
deemed it proper, by this proclamation, to recommend that Thursday the twelfth of January
next be set apart as a day on which all may
have an opportunity of voluntarily offering, at
the same time, in their respective religious*

*assemblies, their humble adoration to the great
Sovereign of the Universe, of confessing their
sins and transgressions, and of strengthening
their vows of repentance and amendment....*

(Appendix no. 14, Volume 11, U.S. Statutes At Large.)

The outcome of this national day of fasting
and prayer presents a historical fulfillment of
God's promise given in Isaiah 65:24: *"And it
shall come to pass, that before they call, I will
answer; and while they are yet speaking, I will
hear."*

Four days before the day set by Madison,
the last battle of this war was fought at New
Orleans, resulting in a victory for the United
States. Peace followed shortly afterwards. As a
result, the two Houses of Congress requested
Madison to proclaim a day of public thanksgiving. The day which he appointed was the second Thursday of April, 1815. The following is
part of his proclamation:

*The Senate and House of Representatives
of the United States, have, by a joint resolution,
signified their desire that a day may be recommended to be observed by the people of the
United States with religious solemnity, as a
day of thanksgiving, and of devout acknowl-
edgments to Almighty God for His great*

goodness manifested in restoring to them the blessing of peace.

No people ought to feel greater obligations to celebrate the goodness of the Great Disposer of events, and of the destiny of nations, than the people of the United States. His kind providence originally conducted them to one of the best portions of the dwelling-place allotted for the great family of the human race. He protected and cherished them, under all the difficulties and trials to which they were exposed in their early days. Under His fostering care, their habits, their sentiments, and their pursuits prepared them for a transition, in due time, to a state of independence and self-government. In the arduous struggle by which it was attained, they were distinguished by multiplied tokens of His benign interposition. During the interval which succeeded, He reared them into the strength and endowed them with the resources which have enabled them to assert their national rights, and to enhance their national character, in another arduous conflict, which is now so happily terminated by a peace and reconciliation with those who have been our enemies....

It is for blessings such as these, and especially for the restoration of the blessing of peace, that I now recommend that the second Thursday in April next, be set apart as a day on

*which the people of every religious denomina-
tion, may, in their solemn assemblies, unite
their hearts and their voices in a free will offering to their heavenly Benefactor, of their hom-
age of thanksgiving, and of their songs of
praise.*

(Appendix no. 16, Volume 11, U.S. Statutes At Large.)

Three Fasts Proclaimed by Lincoln

During the presidency of Abraham Lincoln
three separate days of national humiliation,
prayer and fasting were proclaimed. The prime
cause for each of these was the Civil War, and
the central theme of petition was for the restoration of national peace and unity.

Lincoln's first proclamation was requested
by a joint committee of both Houses of Congress, and the day set apart was the last
Thursday in September, 1861. The following is
part of the proclamation:

*Whereas a joint committee of both Houses
of Congress has waited on the President of the
United States, and requested him to "recommend a day of public Humiliation, Prayer and
Fasting, to be observed by the people of the
United States with religious solemnities, and
the offering of fervent supplications to almighty*

*God for the safety and welfare of these States,
His blessing on their arms, and a speedy restoration of peace."*

*And whereas it is fit and becoming in all
people, at all times, to acknowledge and revere
the Supreme Government of God; to bow in
humble submission to his chastisements; to
confess and deplore their sins and transgressions, in the full conviction that the fear of the
Lord is the beginning of wisdom, and to pray,
with all fervency and contrition, for the pardon
of their past offenses, and for a blessing upon
their present and prospective action....*

*Therefore, I, ABRAHAM LINCOLN,
President of the United States, do appoint the
last Thursday in September next, as a day of
Humiliation, Prayer, and Fasting, for all the
people of the nation. And I do earnestly recommend to all the people, and especially to all
ministers and teachers of religion, of all denominations, and to all heads of families, to
observe and keep that day, according to their
several creeds and modes of worship, in all
humility, and with all religious solemnity, to
the end that the united prayer of the nation may
ascend to the Throne of Grace, and bring down
plentiful blessings upon our Country.*

(Appendix no. 8, Volume 12, U.S. Statutes At Large.)

By specifically including "all heads of families" in his proclamation, Lincoln apparently envisaged prayer and fasting being carried out in the homes of the nation, with parents and children uniting in their worship and petitions. In this, as in other respects, both the language and the spirit of his proclamation are in perfect accord with Scripture.

Lincoln's second proclamation is the one reproduced fully at the beginning of this book.

Lincoln's third proclamation was requested by a concurrent resolution of both Houses of Congress, and the day set apart was the first Thursday of August, 1864. In the closing paragraph of this proclamation, Lincoln made a special plea for the cooperation of all who held positions of authority in every area of national life:

I do hereby further invite and request the heads of the executive departments of this government, together with all legislators, all judges and magistrates, and all other persons exercising authority in the land...and all the other law-abiding people of the United States, to assemble in their preferred places of public worship on that day, and there and then to render to the Almighty and Merciful Ruler of the universe such homages and such confessions, and to offer to Him such supplications as the congress of the United States have...so solemnly, so earnestly, and so reverently recommended.

(Appendix no. 17, Volume 13, U.S. Statutes At Large.)

No claim is here put forward that the above list of public fasting days is in any sense comprehensive or complete. However, combined with the material in our previous chapter about the pilgrims, it suffices to establish one historical fact: **From the beginning of the seventeenth century until at least the second half of the nineteenth century, public days of prayer and fasting played a vital and continuing role in shaping the national destiny of the United States.**

In the light of these official national records, thoughtful Americans should ask of themselves this question: How many of the blessings and the privileges we now enjoy were obtained for us by the prayers of our leaders and governments in previous generations?

Today, as we look back over a little more than three hundred and fifty years of American history, we form the impression of an elaborate pattern, woven out of threads of varying colors and textures. Each thread represents a different background and is associated with differing motives and purposes.

Clear and strong throughout the length of the pattern, we may distinguish one thread of divine purpose. This purpose was born out of the fellowship of the pilgrims and their united prayer and fasting. In each succeeding generation, it has been sustained and continued by the faith, prayers and fasting of like-minded believers. The full and final outworking of this purpose still lies ahead. It is to this that we will devote the final chapter of this book.

12

Climax: The Glorious Church

In the opening chapters of this book, we saw that the church of Jesus Christ, indwelled by the Holy Spirit, is the main representative of God in the earth and the main agent of God's purposes for the world in this age. Later, in chapter 8, we saw that, through the latter rain of the Holy Spirit, God is now restoring the church to His own ordained standards of purity, power, and order. The church, thus restored, will then be enabled to fulfill its God-appointed destiny in the world and to bring to a triumphant climax God's purposes for the close of this age.

Paul's Picture of the Completed Church

In his letter to the Ephesians, Paul describes how the church will be brought to completion and what it will be like when it is complete. In Ephesians 1:22-23, he tells us that the church is Christ's body, and that Christ is the sole and sovereign Head over this body. Then in chapter 4, Paul lists the main ministries given by Christ to His church and the purpose for which they are given:

> *And he gave some, apostles; and some, prophets; and some, evangelists; and some, pastors and teachers;*
> *For the perfecting of the saints, for the work of the ministry, for the edifying of the body of Christ:*
> *Till we all come in the unity of the faith, and of the knowledge of the Son of God, unto a perfect man, unto the measure of the stature of the fullness of Christ.*
> *(Ephesians 4:11-13)*

The five main ministries in the church are listed in verse 11: apostles, prophets, evangelists, pastors and teachers. Verse 12 tells us the purpose of these ministries: the edifying, or building up, of the body of Christ. Verse 13 gives four marks of the completed body. This verse may be more literally rendered: *"Until we all come into the unity of the faith, and of the acknowledging of the Son of God, unto a full-grown man, unto the measure of the stature that represents Christ in His fullness."*

Too often we think of the church as being in a static condition. This is not correct. The church is in a condition of growth and development. The opening word of verse 13, *"until,"* indicates that we are moving toward a predetermined end. This is confirmed by the expression *"in*[to] *the unity of the faith."* We are not yet in the unity of the faith. One glance at the various different groups and denominations around us proves this. But we are moving into this unity. The time is coming when all true Christians will be **united in their faith**.

The way that leads into this unity is indicated by Paul's next phrase, *"the* [acknowledging] *of the Son of God."* All the doctrines of the New Testament center in the Person and work of Christ: the doctrine of salvation centers in the Savior; the doctrine of healing centers in the Healer; the doctrine of sanctification centers in the Sanctifier; the doctrine of deliverance centers in the Deliverer; and so on with all the other great doctrines of Christianity. The true and full expression of each doctrine is in the Person and work of Christ. History has demonstrated that Christians do not achieve unity by discussing doctrine in the abstract. But as Christians are willing to acknowledge Christ in His fullness, and to **give Christ His rightful position in their lives and in the church**, the various doctrines of Christianity all fit together in Him, just like the spokes of a wheel fitting into its hub. Thus the way *"in*[to] *the unity of the faith"* is through *"the* [acknowledging] *of the Son of God."*

This leads also *"to a* [full-grown] *man."* The church is growing up into **mature** manhood. This man, grown to full stature, will be able to represent Christ in all his fullness. He will be, in the truest sense, the embodiment of Christ. He will constitute the consummation of God's purposes for the church as Christ's body: that is, **the perfect revelation of Christ**. Endowed with every grace, every gift, every ministry, this completed church will present to the world a complete Christ.

In Ephesians chapter 5, Paul fills out his picture of the church at the close of this age. He has already presented the church as Christ's body. In this passage, he presents the church as Christ's bride, comparing Christ's relationship to His church with that of a husband to his wife:

*Husbands, love your wives, even as Christ
also loved the church, and gave himself for
it;
That he might sanctify and cleanse it with
the washing of water by the word.*
                        (Ephesians 5:25-26)

In these verses Paul presents Christ in two
main aspects: first as Redeemer, then as Sanctifier. The means of redemption is the blood of
Christ. The means of sanctification is the Word
of God. Christ first redeemed the church by
His blood, shed on the cross, that He might
thereafter sanctify the church by His Word.
The sanctifying operation of God's Word is
compared to the washing of pure water. It requires both these ministries of Christ to make
the church complete.

This agrees with the picture of Christ presented in 1 John 5:6: *"This is he that came by
water and blood, even Jesus Christ: not by water only, but by water and blood. And it is the
Spirit that beareth witness, because the Spirit is
truth."*

Through His blood, shed on the cross,
Christ is the church's Redeemer. Through the
pure water of God's Word, Christ is the
church's Sanctifier. It is the Holy Spirit that
bears witness to both these aspects of Christ.
In the present *"latter rain"* outpouring, the

Holy Spirit is once again placing all the emphasis of His divine authority upon these two provisions of God for the church: redemption by Christ's blood, and sanctification by God's Word. Both alike are essential for the completion of the church.

In Ephesians 5:27, Paul goes on to describe the results that Christ will accomplish in the church through this double ministry: *"That he might present it to himself a glorious church, not having spot, or wrinkle, or any such thing; but that it should be holy and without blemish."*

The first and most conspicuous feature of the church, as here described, is that it will be **glorious**. That is to say, it will be permeated by God's glory. The word *glory* denotes the personal presence of God, made manifest to human senses. After the deliverance of Israel from Egypt, this glory took the form of a cloud, which overshadowed the tabernacle in the wilderness, and which also filled and illuminated the Holy of Holies within the tabernacle. In like manner, the completed church will be overshadowed, filled, and illuminated by the manifest glory of God. As a result, the church will also be **holy** and **without blemish**.

The church pictured by Paul in Ephesians will be the fulfillment of Christ's prayer to the Father for His disciples in John 17:22: *"And*

the glory which thou gavest me I have given them; that they may be one, even as we are one."
It is the glory that will complete the unity. Conversely, it is the united church that alone can show forth the glory. In the preceding verse Jesus says, *"that the world may believe,"* and in the following verse He says, *"that the world may know."* The united, glorified church will be **Christ's witness** to the whole world.

By combining Paul's picture of the church in Ephesians 4:13 with that in Ephesians 5:27, we arrive at seven distinctive marks of the church at the close of this age:

1. The church will be united in its faith.
2. The church will acknowledge Christ as its Head in every aspect of His Person and work.
3. The church will be full-grown.
4. The completed church will present to the world a complete Christ.
5. The church will be permeated by God's glory.
6. The church will be holy.
7. The church will be without blemish.

Of these seven marks, the first four describe the church as Christ's completed body. The last three describe the church as Christ's completed bride.

Isaiah's Portrait of the End-time Church

This New Testament picture of the church at the close of this age is confirmed by various prophecies of the Old Testament. One of the most striking of these prophecies is found in Isaiah. Against a worldwide background of darkness, distress and confusion, Isaiah portrays the end-time church emerging in glory and power:

So shall they fear the name of the Lord from the west, and his glory from the rising of the sun. When the enemy shall come in like a flood, the Spirit of the Lord shall lift up a standard against him.

And the Redeemer shall come to Zion, and unto them that turn from transgression in Jacob, saith the Lord.

As for me, this is my covenant with them, saith the Lord; My spirit that is upon thee, and my words which I have put in thy mouth, shall not depart out of thy mouth, nor out of the mouth of thy seed, nor out of the mouth of thy seed's seed, saith the Lord, from henceforth and for ever.

Arise, shine; for thy light is come, and the glory of the Lord is risen upon thee.

For, behold, the darkness shall cover the earth, and gross darkness the peoples: but

*the Lord shall arise upon thee, and his
glory shall be seen upon thee.
And* [the nations] *shall come to thy light,
and kings to the brightness of thy rising.
Lift up thine eyes round about, and see: all
they gather themselves together, they come
to thee: thy sons shall come from far, and
thy daughters shall be nursed at thy side.
Then thou shalt see, and flow together, and
thine heart shall fear, and be enlarged; because the abundance of the sea shall be
converted unto thee, the forces* [literally,
wealth] *of the* [nations] *shall come unto
them.* (Isaiah 59:19-21; 60:1-5)

In the first part of verse 19 of chapter 59,
Isaiah declares the end purpose of God, which
is to be achieved through the events that follow: *"So shall they fear the name of the Lord
from the west, and his glory from the rising of
the sun."* There is to be a worldwide demon-
stration of God's glory that will cause awe and
wonder among all nations.

The second half of this verse reveals that
Satan, *"the enemy,"* coming *"in like a flood,"*
will attempt to oppose God's purposes, but
that his opposition will be overcome by the
Holy Spirit. Historically, it is the darkest hour
of man's need that calls forth the mightiest
intervention of God. It is *"where sin abounds"*

that God's grace so *"much more abounds"* (Romans 5:20).

The Holy Spirit is here presented by Isaiah as the Standard Bearer of God's army. Just at the moment when God's people are in danger of being totally scattered and defeated, the Holy Spirit lifts up the divine standard. Encouraged by this evidence that God is coming to their help, the people of God from every direction gather around the uplifted standard and regroup for a fresh offensive.

What is the standard which the Holy Spirit uplifts here? In John 16:13-14, Jesus spoke of the Holy Spirit's coming and declared: *"He shall glorify me."* The Holy Spirit has only one standard to uplift. It is not an institution, nor a denomination, nor a doctrine. It is a Person: *"Jesus Christ the same yesterday, and to-day, and for ever"* (Hebrews 13:8). For every true believer, loyalty to this standard—Jesus Christ—is primary. Every other commitment —to institution, denomination, or doctrine—is secondary. Wherever such believers see Christ truly uplifted by the Holy Spirit, they will gather.

In the decades since World War II, this prophecy in the latter part of Isaiah 59:19 has been exactly fulfilled. First, *"the enemy has come in like a flood."* There has been an unparalleled inundation of Satan's influence and activity in every area of life—religious, moral, social, political. Second, *"the Spirit of the Lord [has] lifted up a standard against him."* Every section of Christendom has begun to experience a sovereign, supernatural visitation of the Holy Spirit. This visitation centers around no institution and no human personality, but only around the Lord Jesus Christ. Around the person of Christ, uplifted by the Holy Spirit, the people of God from every background are now regathering.

Isaiah 59:19-20 describes various effects of this visitation. God's people are turning back to Him in repentance. Christ is working again in His church, bringing redemption and deliverance. He is renewing His covenant and restoring the fullness of His Holy Spirit. Once again, God's people have become His witnesses. With God's Spirit upon them, His Word is being proclaimed through their lips.

All age groups are included in this visitation. It is for parents, children, and children's children. Indeed, there is special emphasis upon the young people. This is the same outpouring that is predicted in Joel 2:28 and Acts 2:17: *"Your sons and your daughters shall prophesy, and your young men shall see visions."*

Nor is this a brief or a temporary visitation. It is *"from henceforth and for ever."* The

Holy Spirit's fullness, now being restored to God's people, will never again be taken from them.

The first two verses of Isaiah chapter 60 emphasize the increasing contrast between the light and the darkness. *"Darkness shall cover the earth, and gross darkness the peoples."* But upon God's people the light and glory of His presence will shine forth all the more brightly in the surrounding darkness. The darkness is growing darker, but the light is growing brighter. This is the hour of decision, the parting of the ways. There can be no more neutrality, no more compromise; *"for what fellowship hath righteousness with unrighteousness? and what communion hath light with darkness?"* (2 Corinthians 6:14).

In verse 3, Isaiah describes the impact produced upon the world by the manifestation of the church in its glory. Nations and their rulers will turn and seek for help. Of this hour Jesus spoke in Luke 21:25: *"distress of nations, with perplexity."* The multiplying problems of recent decades have brought the rulers of the nations to the point where they no longer claim to have the solutions. Therefore, whole nations will turn to Christ as He reveals His wisdom and His power through the church.

In chapter 60, verse 4, Isaiah challenges the church to look out over the great influx of people that is coming in. Here again, we see particular emphasis upon the young people: *"thy sons"* and *"thy daughters."*

Verse 5 brings this part of the prophecy to its climax. *"Thou shalt see, and flow together."* The vision of what God is doing will bring His people together. From every historical background and from every section of Christendom, the streams of revival will flow, finally uniting themselves into a single irresistible river. *"Thine heart shall fear, and be enlarged."* Holy awe will come over God's people at the revelation of His power and glory. Yet there will be also an enlargement of heart—an enlarged capacity to comprehend and to fulfill the purposes of God.

To God's people thus regathered, united, and empowered, there will be made available vast financial and material resources: *"the abundance of the sea"* and *"the wealth of the nations."* God has these resources reserved and set aside for the final task which the church has to fulfill.

The Last Great Task

In Matthew 24:3, the disciples asked Jesus a question: *"What shall be the sign of thy coming and of the close of the age?"* (RSV). Their question was specific. They did not ask for signs in the plural, but for the sign—the one final, definite indication that the close of the age was at hand.

In verses 5 through 13, Jesus gave them various signs—various events or trends that would characterize the closing period. However, it was not until verse 14 that He actually answered their specific question: *"And this gospel of the kingdom shall be preached in all the world for a witness unto all nations; and then shall the end come."*

Here is a specific answer to a specific question. When shall the end come? When this Gospel of the kingdom shall have been preached in all the world and to all nations. This confirms a theme that has been emphasized throughout this book: **The initiative in world affairs is with God and His people**. The climax of the age will not be brought about by the actions of secular government or military power, nor by the floods of satanic deception and lawlessness. The final decisive activity will be the preaching of the Gospel of the kingdom. This is a task that can be accomplished only by the church of Jesus Christ.

Scripture is very precise about the message that is to be preached. It is to be *"this gospel of the kingdom."* This is the same message that was preached by Christ and the first disciples. It sets forth Christ in His kingly victory and power. *"Where the word of a king is, there is power"* (Ecclesiastes 8:4). *"For the kingdom of God is not in word, but in power"* (1 Corinthians 4:20). The kingdom Gospel is supernaturally attested *"with signs and wonders, and with divers miracles, and gifts of the Holy Ghost"* (Hebrews 2:4). It will be a true and effective *"witness unto all nations."*

Today the scene is set for the last great act of the church's drama. For the first time in human history, the task of bringing the kingdom Gospel to all nations can be fulfilled within a single generation. Technology has provided both the means of travel and the media of communication which are needed. The cost of utilizing these resources will be tremendous, but in Isaiah 60:5 God has promised to the end-time church *"the abundance of the sea"* and *"the wealth of the nations."* These are His appointed means of provision. The financial and technological resources of the nations are to be made available to the church for the fulfillment of its final task on earth.

At the same time, the latter rain of the Holy Spirit is bringing forth, as Joel promised, a dedicated army of young men and women, ready to fulfill the commission of Jesus in Acts 1:8: *"But ye shall receive power, after that the Holy Spirit is come upon you: and ye shall be witnesses unto me...unto the uttermost part of the earth.*" This is the generation to which David looked forward in Psalm 22:30: *"A seed shall serve him; it shall be accounted to the Lord for a generation."* It is also the period of which Jesus spoke in Matthew 24:34: *"This generation shall not pass, till all these things be fulfilled."*

For the final outworking of His purposes God is thus bringing together the various resources that are needed: the human resources of Spirit-filled young people, and the material resources of wealth and technology. In both these respects, the United States has a unique contribution to make. The first mass outpouring of the Holy Spirit upon today's youth has taken place in the United States and is still proceeding across the nation. At the same time, the financial and technological resources of the United States are the greatest in the modern world. The nation that first placed men on the moon is uniquely qualified to place the messengers of the kingdom Gospel in every nation on earth. By the combined offering of its resources—both human and material—for the worldwide proclamation of the kingdom Gospel, the United Stales will complete the thread of divine destiny that has run through its history for three-and-a-half centuries.

This special purpose of God for the United States was born out of the fellowship of the pilgrims. The vision God gave them was for the restoration of the church. To this they devoted themselves with labor and sacrifice, with prayer and fasting. Today those who share the pilgrims' vision can see its fulfillment approaching. The church of Jesus Christ stands poised to carry the Gospel of the kingdom to all nations on earth. Through the achievement of this final task the church will itself be brought to completion.

From the study of the Scriptures, the pilgrims learned two great truths which they have in turn bequeathed to their spiritual descendants in their own and other lands. First, **the end-time purpose of God is the restoration and completion of the church**. Second, **the source of power for the achievement of this purpose is united prayer and fasting**.

Background of the Author

Derek Prince was born in India of British parents. He was educated as a scholar of Greek and Latin at two of Britain's most famous educational institutions—Eton College and Cambridge University. From 1940 to 1949, he held a Fellowship (equivalent to a resident professorship) in Ancient and Modern Philosophy at King's College, Cambridge. He also studied Hebrew and Aramaic, both at Cambridge University and at the Hebrew University in Jerusalem. In addition, he speaks a number of other modern languages.

In the early years of World War II, while serving as a hospital attendant with the British Army, Derek Prince experienced a life-changing encounter with Jesus Christ, concerning which he writes:

Out of this encounter, I formed two conclusions which I have never since had reason to change: first, that Jesus Christ is alive; second, that the Bible is a true, relevant, up-to-date book. These two conclusions radically and permanently altered the whole course of my life.

At the end of World War II, he remained where the British Army had placed him—in Jerusalem. Through his marriage to his first wife, Lydia, he became father to the eight adopted girls in Lydia's children's home there. Together the family saw the rebirth of the State of Israel in 1948. While serving as educator in Kenya, Derek and Lydia Prince adopted their ninth child, an African baby girl. Lydia died in 1975, and Derek Prince remarried in October 1978. He met his second wife, Ruth, like his first, while she was serving the Lord in Jerusalem. Ruth's three children bring Derek Prince's family to a total of twelve, with many grandchildren and great-grandchildren.

Derek Prince's non-denominational, non-sectarian approach has opened doors for his teaching to people from many different racial and religious backgrounds, and he is internationally recognized as one of the leading Bible expositors of our time. His daily radio broadcast, Today With Derek Prince, reaches more than half the globe including translations into Arabic, five Chinese languages (Mandarin, Amoy, Cantonese, Shanghaiese, Swatow),

Mongolian, Spanish, Russian and Tongan. He has published more than 30 books, which have been translated into more than 50 foreign languages.

Through the Global Outreach Leaders Program of Derek Prince Ministries, his books and audio cassettes are sent free of charge to hundreds of national Christian leaders in the Third World, Eastern Europe and Russia. Now past the age of 75, he still travels the world—imparting God's revealed truth, praying for the sick and afflicted, and sharing his prophetic insight into world event in the light of Scripture.

The international base of Derek Prince Ministries is located in Charlotte, North Carolina, with branch offices in Australia, Canada, Germany, Holland, New Zealand, South Africa, and the United Kingdom.